GET THE SUGAR OUT

GET THE SUGAR OUT

**501 Simple Ways to Cut the Sugar
Out of Any Diet**

Ann Louise Gittleman, M.S., C.N.S.

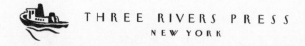

THREE RIVERS PRESS
NEW YORK

Permissions to reprint already published recipes
appear on pages 175–180.

Published by Three Rivers Press, New York, New York.
Member of the Crown Publishing Group.

Random House, Inc. New York, Toronto, London, Sydney, Auckland
www.randomhouse.com

THREE RIVERS PRESS is a registered trademark and the Three Rivers Press
colophon is a trademark of Random House, Inc.

Printed in the United States of America

Design by M. Kristen Bearse

Library of Congress Cataloging-in-Publication Data
Gittleman, Ann Louise.
Get the sugar out : 501 simple ways to cut the sugar out of any diet / by
Ann Louise Gittleman.—1st paperback edition.
Includes bibliographical references and index.
1. Sugar-free diet.   I. Title.
RM237.85.G55   1996   613.2'8—dc20   96-1142

ISBN 0-517-88653-7

20 19 18 17 16 15 14 13

This book is dedicated to
Isaac Aaron Gittleman,
a beloved addition to the
Gittleman family.

CONTENTS

ACKNOWLEDGMENTS

My most profound thanks go to Melissa Diane Smith, whose diligence, research, and commitment to this project made *Get the Sugar Out* possible. Melissa shares my vision of a low-sugar America.

In addition, I would be remiss if I did not personally thank both Helen Smith and Stuart Sandler. Helen provided both practical and literary advice, while Stuart's computer expertise improved this book immeasurably.

Thanks also to Holly Sollars for her recipes, recipe revisions, and tip suggestions. And a big debt of gratitude to Kathryn Arnold and the staff of *Delicious Magazine,* who featured articles about this book before its publication.

It is my profound hope that all the sugar researchers before me are vindicated by this book. I think that experts like William Dufty, Cass Ingram, M.D., Robert Atkins, M.D., and John Yudkin, M.D., would be proud.

PREFACE

The Facts About Sugar

All of us should be eating less sugar. That's probably big news for those of you who thought fat was the Bad Guy. The fact is that ever since we started slashing the fat and consuming those monstrous low-fat muffins and boxes of fat-free cookies and candy, we have actually gotten fatter. Why? Because Americans have been consuming these goodies with abandon, disregarding the fact that they usually have *more* sugar, and sometimes only slightly fewer calories, than the original products.

Take Nabisco Fig Newtons, for example. Two of the original Fig Newtons supply you with 13 grams of sugars and 110 calories. If you eat two Nabisco Fat-Free Fig Newtons, thinking you're doing your body such a favor, you'll get no fat, but you'll get more sugar—15 grams instead of 13 grams—and only 10 fewer calories. What's worse is that the fat in the original cookie helps satiate your appetite so you are apt to eat only a few. With the fat-free kind, people sometimes eat whole boxes without ever feeling satisfied.

Nonetheless, sales of fat-free products have skyrocketed. SnackWell's, a line of reduced-fat cookies and crackers, now outsells Oreo cookies, previously the country's favorite. With the use of these fat-free products, our fat consumption may be going down but our waistlines are expanding. During the last decade, Americans have reduced their fat intake at least 2 percent, but we have also become 30 percent more overweight in almost the same time.

The answer to our battle of the bulge and current health problems then is *not to avoid all fat.* I have written an entire book called *Beyond Pritikin* on how the right type of fat can help promote weight loss and health. The right kind of fat is an essential nutrient that our bodies need. Sugar, on the other hand, is *something we don't need at all.*

Statistics in France seem to prove this. Even though the French diet is higher in fat than the American diet, the French are much less afflicted by obesity and heart disease than Americans are. What's the French secret to maintaining weight and better health? It appears to be because French per capita sugar consumption is *five and a half times less* than that in America (*Hippocrates,* May/June 1990). Humans don't require sugar, yet average Americans consume their body weight in sugar each year.

If all Americans knew the dangers of sugar, it would be withdrawn from our list of food additives. Refined sugar acts more like a drug that our bodies need to detoxify rather than a nutrient-supplying food. Refined sugar is, in fact, nutrient-less. Important nutrients such as chromium, manganese, cobalt, copper, zinc, and magnesium are stripped away in sugar refining, and our bodies actually have to use their own mineral reserves just to digest it. With lots of calories but no nutrients, sugar is the number one cause of America's weight problem and lack of nutrition—a combination known as *overconsumptive malnutrition.* What this term basically means is that Americans are consuming too many calories that add up in weight but don't give us the nutrients we need to keep our bodies functioning properly.

Our distant ancestors ate no concentrated sugars. Even in the infancy of this country, people ate sugar only as a rare treat. But now sugar and other sweeteners have become part of our everyday diet. Little by little, as our country has developed and become more "civilized," Americans have become more and more "sugarized." The following chart shows the alarming rise in sugar consumption in America since the early 1800s.

Sugar Consumption per Person Each Year

YEAR	AMOUNT IN POUNDS
Early 1800s	12
1850	22
1875	41
1895	63
1915	95
1935	115
1955	119
1976	125
1990	130–40

Source: Miller, Bruce, D.D.S., and James Scala, Ph.D., *Better Health* (Dallas, Texas: Miller Enterprises, Inc., 1994).

And things have gotten worse since 1990. At last count, Americans consumed *152 pounds of sweeteners per year,* and when you add noncaloric sweeteners to that number, it was almost 165 pounds. Compare that to the consumption of less than 10 pounds of sugar per year in the late 1700s and you can see that *sugar consumption has risen more than 1,500 percent in the last two hundred years!*

Such a drastic change in the human diet in less than two centuries is a cause for great concern. Evolutionary changes occur over hundreds of thousands of years; the human body of today is still very similar to the Stone Age model of forty thousand years ago. To change the kinds of calories consumed by humans so dramatically in so short a time is an invitation to trouble. Our bodies simply haven't had time to respond and adapt to this nutrient-poor source of calories—and it appears that our bodies are rebelling with a multitude of physical ailments, telling us loudly and clearly that they don't like what they're being fed.

We all know sugar causes dental cavities, but recent evidence has shown that sugar is associated with weakened immunity, heart disease, high blood pressure, cancer, and more. (For a complete list of the ailments associated with sugar consumption, see "The Problems with Sugar," page xxii.) We also know without a doubt that excess calories from sugar can turn into body fat just like excess calories from fat can. Remember that the next time you want to think that *fat-free* means "eat all you want."

Some of you might already be well aware that sugar is harmful to your health and be eager to move on to the tips. If you are, let me get to the bottom line: Fat, like protein, is an essential nutrient for human health. *Simple sugars are not!* We could live very nicely (much better, in fact) if we never ate another ounce of sugar.

If you would like to understand the intricate details of *why* that statement is true, keep on reading. If you do decide to skip the next section and move directly on to the tips right now, I recommend that you come back to the important information that follows when you have more time. Knowing exactly why we should avoid sugar helps instill a much deeper resolve to reduce our sugar intake than if we don't know.

UNDERSTANDING SUGAR

The term *sugar* can be misleading.

Most of us hear the word and think of table sugar, the end product of the refining of sugarcane. But the term can be used in so many different contexts and have so many different meanings that confusion abounds. (Food manufacturers couldn't be happier about this confusion because they often use it to their advantage.)

To understand what sugar really is, you first have to understand some basics about carbohydrates. Carbohydrates are one of three energy-producing nutrients our bodies need; the other two are protein and fat. As a fuel, carbohydrates are the cleanest burning of the three and the best provider of glucose, a fuel our muscles need for get-up-and-go and a fuel our brains need for clear thinking and steady behavior.

There are two significantly different types of carbohydrates —simple and complex. Simple carbohydrates, which consist of one or two sugar units in every molecule, are also known as *simple sugars*. They supply virtually instant energy for the body, but they don't provide energy that lasts. As you might have guessed, *table sugar* (also known as dextrose or sucrose) is one type of simple sugar. But so are *natural sweeteners* like honey and molasses; *fructose,* which is found naturally in fruits and can also be a sweetener; and *lactose,* which is a naturally occurring sugar found in dairy products. (For a complete list of different types of simple sugars, see tip 79.)

Complex carbohydrates, on the other hand, are made up of long chains of simple sugars. As their name implies, they are much more complex in structure than simple sugars and require longer digestion to be absorbed. This is beneficial in the long run because the sugars they contain are released more slowly and gradually in the bloodstream, supplying steadier, longer-lasting energy for the body. Complex carbohydrates are found in *starches* (such as whole grains and starchy vegetables such as potatoes), *legumes* (such as beans and peas), and *vegetables* (such as lettuce, broccoli, and zucchini).

When most people hear of the value of carbohydrates in the diet, they make little distinction between the two kinds. Avoiding vegetables and munching on sugar-laden muffins, cookies, and candy, even if they are "low-fat," is not the way we should meet our carbohydrate needs, yet it is the way more and more of us are choosing to eat. At the beginning of this century, two-thirds of the carbohydrates eaten by Americans came from complex sources such as potatoes, vegetables, and grains. *Today, amazingly, half of all carbohydrates consumed come from simple sugars.* These statistics confirm what we already know: We are becoming sugarholics.

What the statistics don't show, however, is equally important to understand. Most of the "complex" carbohydrates Americans consume aren't really that complex after all. Although classified as complex carbohydrates (because they're made from grains, not sugars), pasta, bread, and bagels really react more like simple sugars in the body because they're highly refined. In refining, nutrient- and fiber-rich whole grains are converted into processed foods that have a long shelf life, but many calories and few nutrients (sometimes as much as *86 percent less of some nutrients than are in the original grain*). Nutritionally, there is little difference between processed carbohydrates and simple sugars. In fact, far from being healthy foods, these processed carbohydrates contribute to blood-sugar, weight, and malnutrition problems and give us little in return. You should think of processed carbohydrates as hidden sugars in the diet. (They're "hidden" because they are disguised as complex carbohydrates.)

When either sugars or processed carbohydrates are eaten, they are broken down almost immediately, and a flood of sugar is released directly into the bloodstream. In response to so much sugar, the pancreas secretes insulin, a hormone that is designed to restore blood-sugar equilibrium by taking excess sugar out of the bloodstream and either moving it into muscle glycogen for energy for our muscles or moving it into fat storage. But the human body was never designed to deal with so many concentrated sweeteners, so the pancreas ends up doing its job "too well." In response to excess sugar in the bloodstream, the pancreas produces so much insulin that blood sugar drops too low. The result is a quick burst of energy followed by an equally fast drop in energy. At the same time, insulin causes sugar removed from the bloodstream to be *stored as body fat* instead. Once you understand these basic nutrition principles, you can see how America's obsession with fat-free (but sugar- and processed-carbohydrate-rich) goodies is *not* the way to lose weight or to provide any kind of long-term energy.

To understand sugars and carbohydrates and the insulin response to them, it's also extremely helpful to know about the Glycemic Index of foods. The Glycemic Index is a listing based upon real-life blood-sugar levels after the ingestion of various foods. Low-glycemic foods rank between 0 and 40 on the scale and raise the blood sugar slowly and gradually. They are the least likely to cause blood-sugar fluctuations, followed, of course, by moderate-glycemic foods. High-glycemic foods, however, cause an alarmingly fast rise in blood sugar, followed by an equally severe blood-sugar crash. In other words, they are high inducers of insulin.

The following chart is the Glycemic Index from my revised *Beyond Pritikin,* which will help you get to know foods in terms of their glycemic rating.

THE GLYCEMIC
INDEX OF FOODS

RAPID INDUCERS OF INSULIN

Glycemic index greater than 100 percent
Puffed rice
Corn flakes
Maltose
Puffed wheat
French baguette
Instant white rice
40% bran flakes
Rice Krispies
Weetabix
Tofu ice-cream substitute
Millet

Glycemic index of 100 percent
Glucose
White bread
Whole-wheat bread

Glycemic index between 90 and 99 percent
Grape-Nuts
Carrots
Parsnips
Barley (whole-meal)
Muesli
Shredded wheat
Apricots
Corn chips

Glycemic index between 80 and 89 percent
Rolled oats
Oat bran
Honey
White rice
Brown rice
White potato
Corn
Rye (whole-meal)
Shortbread
Ripe banana
Ripe mango
Ripe papaya

Glycemic index between 70 and 79 percent
All-Bran
Kidney beans
Wheat (coarse)
Buckwheat
Oatmeal cookies

MODERATE INDUCERS OF INSULIN

Glycemic index between 60 and 69 percent
Raisins
Mars candy bar
Spaghetti (white)
Spaghetti (whole-wheat)
Pinto beans
Macaroni
Rye (pumpernickel)
Bulgur
Couscous
Wheat kernels

Beets
Apple juice
Applesauce

Glycemic index between 50 and 59 percent
Potato chips
Barley
Green banana
Lactose
Peas (frozen)
Sucrose
Yam
Custard
Dried white beans

Glycemic index between 40 and 49 percent
Sweet potato
Navy beans
Peas (dried)
Bran
Lima beans
Rye (whole-grain)
Oatmeal (steel-cut)
Sponge cake
Butter beans
Grapes
Oranges
Orange juice

REDUCED INSULIN SECRETION

Glycemic index between 30 and 39 percent
Apples
Pears
Tomato soup

Ice cream
Black-eyed peas
Chickpeas
Milk (skim)
Milk (whole)
Yogurt
Fish sticks (breaded)

Glycemic index between 20 and 29 percent
Lentils
Fructose
Plums
Peaches
Grapefruit
Cherries

Glycemic index between 10 and 19 percent
Soybeans
Peanuts

After looking over the Glycemic Index, keep in mind three things:

1. Foods that rank lower on the index help maintain weight, balance blood sugar, and give better, longer-term energy than higher-index foods, which give quick bursts of energy.

2. Eating some protein or fat with moderate- or high-glycemic foods helps to slow down the body's insulin response and keep blood sugar more steady.

3. Even when they rank equal to whole-grain products on the Glycemic Index, processed carbohydrates such as white pasta are still less desirable than whole-grain products because they lack vitamins, minerals, and fiber.

Once you understand the structure and different kinds of sugar, and the body's glycemic response, you can understand why sugar harms your health.

THE PROBLEMS WITH SUGAR

Sugar has been blamed for nearly every known disease and even for the fall of several empires. While those accusations may sound like exaggerations, they probably are closer to the truth than you realize.

Saying sugar is bad for you is the ultimate understatement. The far-reaching problems sugar can cause are well documented in medical journals throughout the world, and new sugar-disease connections are made each year.

Even as far back as the late 1960s and early 1970s—before I received my master's degree in nutrition—nutritional pioneers such as Adelle Davis, Carlton Fredericks, Dr. Herman Goodman, Dr. T. L. Cleave, and Dr. John Yudkin were already warning the public about the dangers of eating too much refined sugar. Twenty years earlier, E. M. Abrahamson, M.D., and A. W. Pezet wrote about the insulin connection to disease, the result of too much sugar in the diet.

This information, a basic part of my nutrition training, never found its way to the American public. It got lost in the 1980s amidst the outcries that all fat was bad. Americans ended up blaming fat for their health problems instead of sugar, and since then, the health problems of Americans have not lessened but have, in fact, worsened.

Take, for example, heart disease, cancer, and diabetes—the three leading disease killers in the United States today.

Although the media have presented dietary fat as the villain in the development of these diseases, sugar appears to be the real culprit.

CARDIOVASCULAR DISEASE The sugar connection to coronary-artery and heart disease was noticed in the 1970s. In the classic study *The Saccharine Disease* (Keats Publishing, 1975), surgeon Capt. T. L. Cleave showed convincing evidence that increases in cardiovascular disease, diabetes, and other common diseases could be traced to increases in sugar and refined-carbohydrate intake. These diseases were virtually nonexistent in primitive cultures, he noted, *until about twenty years after the societies began eating refined carbohydrates.*

British researcher John Yudkin, M.D., came to a similar conclusion. In his book *Sweet and Dangerous* (Wyden Books, 1972), Dr. Yudkin cited numerous examples in a variety of societies that showed that *sugar was a more likely cause of heart disease than fat.* For example, the Masai and Sumburu tribes of East Africa, he explained, have almost no heart disease, yet they eat a high-fat diet of mostly meat and milk but no sugar.

Recent research is proving the validity of the theories posed by Drs. Cleave and Yudkin, showing a direct relationship between sugar and heart disease because of insulin. Remember that when sugar is eaten, insulin is produced. Insulin not only helps to store excess sugar as fat (as explained before), but also helps regulate blood triglyceride levels, which are a major predictor of the development of heart disease. The more sugar you eat, the more insulin your pancreas will produce, and the higher your triglyceride levels are likely to be.

High insulin levels in the blood are also linked to low levels of HDL cholesterol (the "good" cholesterol), high blood pressure, and obesity—three other important heart-disease risk factors. Caused by the common problem of insulin resistance, this conglomeration of symptoms has been named Syndrome X by insulin researcher Dr. Gerald Reaven, and it seems to be affecting a growing number of Americans. It's important to note that even though America's fat intake has recently gone down, our intake of sugars and refined starches has shot up, and our incidence of heart disease is continuing to climb.

CANCER   As with heart disease, the prevalence of cancer has dramatically increased as America's (and other societies') sugar consumption has risen. While it's not clear whether sugar actually causes healthy cells to mutate and become cancerous, we do know one thing for sure: *Once cells become cancerous, they feed directly on sugar,* like a fermenting yeast organism, and *sugar can accelerate tumor growth.* As already noted, Americans consume on average 152 pounds of sugar per person each year and often experience erratic blood-sugar swings. "This constant intravenous fusion of cancer fuel is a primary reason for our cancer incidence," Patrick Quillin, Ph.D., R.D., wrote in his recent book *Beating Cancer with Nutrition* (Nutrition Times Press, 1994). "Elevating blood glucose in a cancer patient is like throwing gasoline on a smoldering fire," Dr. Quillin warned, so eating foods that promote balanced blood sugar is advisable for individuals who have cancer and, as a preventive measure, for those who don't.

ADULT-ONSET DIABETES   Adult-onset diabetes, also known as type II diabetes, is another degenerative disease that has increased in frequency as sugar consumption has increased. Sugar's connection to this disease seems clear: During World War II, when sugar consumption in the United States dropped, the number of cases of adult-onset diabetes also dropped sharply.

This form of diabetes accounts for 98 percent of all the diabetes cases in America today and is considered to be almost entirely diet-related. It develops when insulin receptors in the cells no longer respond to the insulin being produced by the pancreas, and the cells are less able to get energy from the food we eat. Excess calories are then converted to fat, and numerous serious health complications can develop. Most health professionals agree that too many sugars and refined carbohydrates are at least a major contributing factor in the disease.

HYPOGLYCEMIA Though diabetes is caused by high blood sugar, hypoglycemia is low blood sugar, a condition that often precedes the development of adult-onset diabetes. In hypoglycemia, the pancreas reacts to excess processed carbohydrates in the diet by sending out so much insulin that blood sugar drops too low, resulting in fatigue, lack of concentration, anxiety, moods swings, and irritability. Several health professionals, such as research psychologist Alexander Schauss, Ph.D., believe that alcoholics and drug addicts start out as hypoglycemics first and that hypoglycemia can also lead to criminal activity. Since almost all Americans eat too much sugar, many nutritionists think that most Americans are on an almost certain collision course with this disease.

IMPAIRED IMMUNITY Sugar is a known immunosuppressant. This is frightening considering that our ability to withstand all diseases (from the common cold to AIDS) depends on having an active, healthy immune system. No matter what form it takes, sugar paralyzes the immune system in a variety of ways:

1. It has been proven to destroy the germ-killing ability of white blood cells for up to five hours after ingestion.
2. It reduces the production of antibodies, proteins that combine with and inactivate foreign invaders in the body.

3. It interferes with the transport of vitamin C, one of the most important nutrients for all facets of immune function.

4. It causes mineral imbalances and sometimes allergic reactions, both of which weaken the immune system.

5. It neutralizes the action of essential fatty acids, thus making cells more permeable to invasion by allergens and microorganisms.

OTHER HEALTH PROBLEMS   As if this were not evidence enough to get the sugar out of your diet, it's only the tip of the iceberg. Excessive sugar consumption is believed to cause or at least contribute to all of the symptoms, deficiencies, and ailments in the list below. This list was compiled from a detailed review of hundreds of books, articles, and scientific studies that I have researched over the past twenty years.

SUGAR-RELATED AILMENTS

Acne

Addictions to drugs,
    caffeine & food

Adrenal gland exhaustion

Alcoholism

Allergies

Anxiety

Appendicitis

Arthritis

Asthma

Behavior problems

Binge eating

Bloating

Bone loss

Cancer
    (particularly breast cancer
    & colon/rectal cancer)

Candidiasis

Cataracts

Colitis

Constipation

Depression

Dermatitis

Diabetes

Difficulty concentrating

Diverticulitis &
    diverticulosis

Eczema

Edema
Emotional problems
Endocrine gland
   dysfunction
Fatigue
Food cravings
Gallstones
Gout
Heart Disease
High blood cholesterol
High estrogen levels
High triglyceride levels
Hormonal problems
Hyperactivity
Hypertension
   (high blood pressure)
Hypoglycemia
Impaired digestion of all
   foods
Indigestion
Insomnia
Kidney stones

Liver dysfunction
Liver enlargement & fatty
   liver syndrome
Low HDL cholesterol
Menstrual difficulties
Mental illness
Mood swings
Muscle pain
Nearsightedness
Obesity
Osteoporosis
Overacidity
Parasitic infections
Premature aging & wrinkles
Premenstrual syndrome
Psoriasis
Rheumatism
Shortened life span
Tooth decay
Ulcers
Vaginal yeast infections
Weakened immunity

When I see this list, I find it as overwhelming as you probably do—and I've been looking at the evidence against sugar for more than twenty years!

But no matter how difficult it is to realize that something so sweet can really be a devil in disguise, we have to start believing it. The hard facts are staring us in the face and telling us in no uncertain terms that our health and lives depend upon it.

HOW MUCH SUGAR DO WE NEED?

Our bodies do not need simple sugars at all.

As amazing as that may sound, here are the facts: The human body needs *about two teaspoons of sugar* in the bloodstream at any one time. That small amount can easily be met through the digestion of complex carbohydrates, protein, and fat. And those complex carbohydrates don't even need to include fruit. We can meet our sugar requirements quite adequately from vegetables, legumes, and grains. (As surprising as that may be, it's true. In fact, some individuals, such as those afflicted with serious yeast infections or those with very high triglyceride levels, need to avoid fruit until their conditions improve. The sugar in fruit feeds yeasts and also raises triglyceride levels just as refined sugar does.)

While most of us do not need to eliminate fruit from our diets, we do need to avoid refined sugar at all costs. Nutritionist Nancy Appleton, Ph.D., explained why in her book *Lick the Sugar Habit* (Avery Publishing, 1988): "Even if we were to eat no sugar at all, our bodies would still have plenty of sugar. Every teaspoon of refined sugar you eat works to throw the body out of balance and compromise its health."

At this point, you may be saying to yourself, "But I have a sweet tooth. If I shouldn't eat refined sugar, what can I eat to satisfy that sweet tooth?" The answer is simple: fresh vegetables and fruits.

We have to remember that nature provided us with all the sugar we require in vegetables and fruits. These foods also provide the fiber and nutrients we need to properly utilize the sugars they contain. In addition, vegetables and fruits supply powerful, immune-boosting chemicals and antioxidants, some of our best allies to help fight off disease. All of these benefits make vegetables and fruits the only sources of sugars we should regularly include in our daily diets.

SO WHAT DO WE EAT?

Once you start realizing how many foods have added sugars and sweeteners, you might ask yourself, "Just what in the world can I eat?"

Before your throw up your hands in despair, let me assure you that you still have plenty of delicious and totally satisfying food options. Low-sugar eating will not leave you wanting as long as you let go of misconceptions about nutrition, such as the claim that all meats and fats are bad for you. Quite to the contrary, protein and essential fatty acids are required to keep your blood sugar balanced. And blood-sugar equilibrium, it turns out, is one of the most important but often overlooked keys to health.

We know that too much protein and fat in the diet can cause health problems (just as too little of these nutrients can). We have also learned recently that too many carbohydrates can cause disease. So what's the answer? What constitutes the optimal diet?

The answer is surprisingly simple. *The optimal diet should be balanced.* It should contain sufficient protein from both animal and vegetable sources to help support our bodies' tissue growth and repair, immune integrity, fluid balance, digestive enzyme function, and metabolism. It should contain adequate complex carbohydrates from vegetables, fruits, whole grains, and legumes to give us the best kind of fuel for our muscles and brain functions, and fiber to keep our digestive tracts healthy. And the optimal diet also needs to have sufficient high-quality fat in the form of expeller-pressed oils, nuts, and seeds to help balance blood sugar, strengthen cell and mucous membrane integrity, and provide long-term energy. Ideally, each meal or snack should have an almost equal balance of these three nutrients.

Eating in a balanced way helps promote optimal blood-sugar levels. More and more evidence is showing that maintaining balanced blood-sugar levels will help you function at your very best. When your blood-sugar level is stable, you have extended energy, balanced moods, and greater mental focus and attention. And don't forget that you lessen your risks of developing any of the diseases to which excessive sugar consumption has been linked.

As we know by now, refined sugar should not be a component of the optimal diet. This is becoming glaringly evident. Even the recently developed Food Guide Pyramid warns Americans to limit their sugar consumption.

Since getting sugar out of the diet is vital for good health, your first step must be to get refined sweeteners out of the basic foods you eat every day. At first, this seems almost impossible, until you realize that most of the sugars Americans eat come from processed foods. Once you eliminate those sources of hidden sugars and eat natural foods as your ancestors did, excessive sugar is no longer much of a problem. The guidelines are really pretty simple: Stick to lean meats, fish, eggs, legumes, nuts, whole grains, and vegetables in the entrées and snacks you eat. Once you do this, your diet as a whole becomes low in sugar and you will be able to afford a nutrient-rich sweet treat from time to time without suffering ill effects.

It's natural to have a sweet tooth. After all, the first food we consume—mother's milk—is naturally sweet and so are fruits and vegetables. The key to satisfying your sweet tooth without experiencing sugar's troublesome health risks is to satisfy it naturally and intelligently. This means turning to moderate amounts of more healthful, nutritious sources of sweets that don't deplete your body as refined sugars do. Getting the sugar out of your diet does not necessarily mean taking the sweetness out. Believe it or not, sweet treats can be a part of a healthy diet as long as you use wholesome ingredients (and a little bit of sugar savvy) in your culinary indulgences.

Whether you decide to enjoy small amounts of natural sweets in moderation, eat them only on rare occasions, or avoid them altogether, this book will help you gain control of the role sugar plays in your life. Doing so will help you enjoy the sweet things in life without the bitter consequences.

USING THIS BOOK

Getting the sugar out of your diet involves more than simply passing up dessert.

Sugar is pervasive in our society, not only in obvious forms such as cookies, cakes, and candy, but in just about any other food you can think of. From packaged meats to soups to commercial salt, sugar is in there. It's even hidden in such nonfood items as vitamin and mineral supplements, aspirin, prescription and over-the-counter drugs, and various cosmetics.

Cutting down on sugar has to involve a multifaceted approach. It requires developing a "sugar savvy"—knowing where to watch out for sugar and how to creatively and healthfully live without it.

The tips in this book are designed to help you do just that. You probably won't be willing or able to use all 501 suggestions, but that's okay. Remember that this book was written to give helpful hints for everyone: people just wanting to cut refined sugar out of their diets, diabetics who need to cut almost all forms of sugars out—and everyone in between. Just start using the tips that seem easiest and most appealing to you, and your success with those tips may spur you on to try others. In any case, even if you incorporate only one-tenth of the tips in this book, you're sure to reduce the sugar in your diet and change your life in a positive and noticeable way.

In addition to avoiding processed sugar, getting the sugar out also means avoiding processed carbohydrate products such as white rice and refined white-flour products such as commercial pasta and bread. These foods are so processed, lacking the fiber and most of the nutrients of the original grain, that *they are metabolized just like sugar and almost as fast as sugar.*

All of us should try to avoid eating these foods. The evidence is simply too overwhelming that refined carbohydrates such as these cause nutritional deficiencies, wide swings in blood sugar, and degenerative diseases. The more any food is broken down, the more the food's nutrients and fiber are lost—and the more trouble it causes our blood-sugar-regulating mechanisms.

Refined sugar is a perfect example of this. Although the sugarcane plant has naturally occurring vitamins and minerals, by the time the sugar derived from that plant reaches your sugar bowl, it is essentially a nutrient-void food. In fact, because it supplies you with nothing but empty calories, sugar really acts more like a chemical in the body than a life-giving food. It has been implicated as a causal or contributing factor in some sixty different ailments and diseases, some of which are life-threatening. That's why eliminating refined white sugar is tip number one. It needs to be the top priority in your quest to get the sugar out.

Using natural sweeteners such as the ones mentioned in this book is a relatively easy way to wean yourself from refined sugar, but as you begin replacing sugar with natural sweeteners, remember this: Your ultimate goal should be to reduce the *total* amount of sugars you consume, not simply to exchange white sugar for a more natural sweetener. To help you in this pursuit, I have marked many tips and recipes throughout this book with

Sweet Tooth ratings, ranging from one to three. (Tips without a *Sweet Tooth* rating are simply general concepts you need to understand to develop your sugar savvy, or tips and recipes that satisfy your taste buds in nonsweet ways.)

One Sweet Tooth means that the tips and recipes so marked range from not sweet at all to slightly sweet in nature. Desserts with this rating, for example, will help you satisfy your sweet tooth in a subtle way, which is often all that is needed. Tips with *One Sweet Tooth* either contain *zero to four grams of sugars per serving* or rank *low on the Glycemic Index*, a scale that measures the rate at which different carbohydrates break down to be released as sugar in the bloodstream. Low-glycemic foods release their energy more slowly and steadily and cause less trouble for the body than high-glycemic foods.

I have given *Two Sweet Teeth* to those tips, recipes, or foods that provide *five to eight grams of sugars per serving* and those that contain a combination of foods that together raise your blood-sugar level slightly more than low-glycemic foods—in other words, foods that produce *a moderate response on the Glycemic Index*. These tips and foods are intermediate ways to indulge your yen for sweetness and can usually be tolerated in moderation when you are in good health and when your diet as a whole is low in sugar.

The *Three Sweet Teeth* ranking alerts you to those tips and foods that have *more than eight grams of sugars per serving* or rank *high on the Glycemic Index*. Such foods should only be eaten as rare treats or for special occasions. They can also be used as the means to stop eating white sugar, then eating less sugar altogether. *Three Sweet Teeth*–marked foods are not low in sugars, but they offer a superior alternative to the usual decadent sweets because they are made with healthful sweeteners instead of white sugar. They will satisfy those who feel the need to have an extrasweet dessert from time to time, but they should not be eaten often because they can contribute to weight problems, uneven blood-sugar levels, and all the other health problems often associated with refined sugar. Foods and recipes designated with *Three Sweet Teeth* raise the blood sugar very high and very quickly (and can be followed by an equally severe blood-sugar "crash") when they aren't balanced with some protein and fat to slow down the release of sugar in the bloodstream. If you have trouble giving up sweets, following *Three Sweet Teeth*–marked tips is a good place to start and an important step in the right direction, but I wouldn't be honest if I were to tell you that following this step alone will take you far enough to enjoy your best health.

Also included in this book are Bonus Tips, which are not counted in the 501 tips because they are not specifically about cutting the sugar out of your diet. They will, however, add to your culinary IQ, make things easier in the kitchen, provide valuable nutrition knowledge, or help you toward a new, more interesting way of eating.

Throughout *Get the Sugar Out*, I refer to other books, both as sources of recipes and as references for related topics. Since the relationship between sugar and our health is complex, you may want to refer to these books for more detailed information on topics of interest to you.

In addition to references for further reading, I mention specific brand-name products. As long as you pick them with care, convenience products can help you stick to a lower-sugar way of living. The products I have mentioned are not necessarily the only ones or the absolute best ones in a particular category, but they can be very useful. Of course, not every product will agree with you or your lifestyle, so it's up to you to weed out the products (and tips, for that matter) that aren't helpful to you.

Tolerance for sugars and other carbohydrates is an individual thing. Some people may not seem to have a problem metabolizing sugars and refined carbohydrates, while others do. But no matter how well you're handling sugars now, ingesting high-sugar items day after day and year after year will eventually take its toll on your pancreas and adrenal glands.

If you are not currently having health problems on a high-sugar diet, you're fortunate—and unusual. A growing number of Americans—perhaps half of all adults and a larger percentage of the obese—have abused refined sugars and carbohydrates and are developing not only sugar sensitivity but carbohydrate sensitivity as well. More and more research is showing that sugar and carbohydrate sensitivity is associated with such conditions as obesity, heart disease, and diabetes, to name a few.

Therefore, even if you don't presently have health problems, it's much better for you to make gradual changes and cut down on your sugar level now than to wait until later when your health (and perhaps even your life) might depend on it.

Some of you may have serious conditions that warrant maintenance of extra-strict control over your sugar intake. If you have a weight problem, heart disease, hypoglycemia, diabetes, cancer, yeast problems, parasites, or any condition involving a weak immune system, the evidence is convincing that you should reduce your sugar intake. Individual tolerances do vary, but if you have any of the above conditions, you may even need to avoid natural sugar-rich fruit until your health improves. I only use natural sweeteners in my diet on occasion because I find I feel better mentally, emotionally, and physically on a very low-sugar regime. But that's what's right for me.

How far you go in your sugar-slashing quest is entirely up to you. It will depend on your individual biochemistry, your present health, your willpower, and how well you develop your sugar savvy. Make sure to celebrate each of your successful steps toward achieving your long-term goals, no matter how small it may seem, and I promise the rewards to your health will be well worth your efforts.

The first reward you get is congratulations from me! By reading this book, you are taking a big step: making a commitment to a healthier way of living. Enjoy yourself as you begin your health-enhancing, sugar-lowering adventure!

CHAPTER 1

Get the Sugar Out
of Your Kitchen

Many sugar-cutting tips have multiple uses. Once you learn them, you can use them when making breakfast, lunch, dinner, snacks, and yes, even healthful desserts. They can be utilized time and again until they become habits and maybe even family traditions.

The tips in this chapter are the ones you should begin with. They are fundamental sugar-busters—basic concepts to help you identify sugar in all its various forms and to teach you to limit, substitute for, or eliminate it in the foods you put in your grocery cart, the foods you have in your kitchen, and the way you prepare food.

Start the way that suits you best. Most people like to ease into changes, so begin by remembering the concepts and using the tips that seem most simple and appealing to you. Once those become second nature, you'll be more apt to try some of the others.

Lifestyle changes like cutting the sugar out of your diet have a much better chance of taking root when you know exactly how and why you should make those changes. The tips in this chapter cover those hows and whys and serve as the foundation for all of the other tips in this book. Get to know this chapter well and know that the efforts you are putting in today will pay off in rewards to your health tomorrow.

TOP TEN TIPS

1. ▪ The very easiest way to cut sugar is to stop adding it to foods such as cereal and fruits and to drinks such as herbal tea, coffee, and coffee substitutes. Simply eliminating nutrient-empty processed sugars from your kitchen is a good way to start. This means not only table sugar but granulated sugar, dextrose, raw sugar, turbinado sugar, brown sugar, and powdered sugar as well.

2. ▪ Eliminate processed carbohydrates from your kitchen. Although many people don't realize it, refined carbohydrates such as white rice, white bread, and white pasta are quickly converted to sugars in the body and disrupt the body's blood-sugar and fat-control systems. Keeping these common products out of your home is a simple yet effective way to maintain a better-balanced blood-sugar level.

3. ▪ Stick with unprocessed whole foods. That's the only way to be sure you're greatly reducing your sugar intake. Poultry, meat, fish, and eggs are, of course, sugar-free, and legumes, grains, nuts, vegetables, and fruits, which may have some naturally occurring sugars, are full of nutrients and fiber, two ingredients that help balance blood sugar.

4. ▪ Thin out sweeteners or sweet foods, even natural ones, whenever you can. The idea isn't to substitute one sugar addiction for another one, but to gradually and permanently cut down on all forms of sugar in your diet. Dilute concentrated sweeteners like honey with water and mix sweet foods like granola with unsweet foods such as plain cereal and nuts to reduce the total amount of sugar consumed.

5. ▪ Beware of fat-free foods, those new creations that seem as if they'd be so helpful to us but are actually contributing to America's increasing weight and health problems. "Fat-free" may be in bold letters on the label, but what the manufacturers don't tell you is that the products are sugar rich, sometimes containing two or more times the sugar found in the regular version of that product that naturally contains a little fat. High amounts of sugar not balanced with protein and fat cause the pancreas to release insulin, the body's main fat-storage hormone. Fat-free products may sound good on paper, but in the ultimate irony, fat-free products are helping to make Americans fat.

6. ▪ The more natural the food, the better. It's well established now that the more processed a food is, the more it will tend to raise your blood sugar. Since balanced blood sugar levels are the goal, opt for foods as close to their natural state as possible. Choose an orange in place of orange juice, an apple over applesauce, and brown rice instead of white rice.

7. ▪ Become a food detective. To reduce sugar, you have to know where it is first. To do that, you have to be alert, ask questions, and pay attention to the information you receive about food. Learn to recognize important clues—clues such as how many grams of sugar are listed on a food label, the ingredients in a food, and how sweet a food tastes to you. Once you identify those foods with a high or hidden sugar content, you know them for what they really are: nutrient robbers and troublemakers for your body.

8. ▪ Eat for taste *and* good nutrition, not just taste alone. Your tastes can change after all, but your fundamental nutrient requirements have to be met each and every day. It's far better to have your taste buds rebel for a short while than to have your body break down from nutrient deficiencies. Keep this is mind when you're asked to change long-standing habits for new, healthier, sugar-reducing ways of eating.

9. ▪ Listen to your body. A recent book of mine, *Your Body Knows Best*, goes into this subject in more depth, but just know that your body gives powerful signals about what's right for you even when your taste buds don't want to listen. For example, if you get an initial high after eating a piece of chocolate but two hours later feel lethargic, irritable, and depressed, your body is going to great lengths to tell you something. Try to pick out those foods that make you feel good over the long term—mentally, emotionally, and physically—and you'll make great strides toward stabilizing your blood sugar.

10. ▪ Eat regular, balanced meals. This may sound like old-fashioned advice your mother may have given you, but scientific research is proving its inherent wisdom. Some research indicates that the body operates more efficiently when each meal or snack that you eat contains approximately 40 percent carbohydrates, 30 percent protein, and 30 percent fat. This formula keeps your blood sugar in the optimal zone for as long as four or five hours. Balanced blood-sugar levels mean better concentration, better mood, greater energy and stamina (and therefore less need or temptation to grab something sweet for quick energy).

TRICKS OF THE TRADE

11. ▪ Try an elimination diet, cutting out sugar in all forms (even natural sweeteners such as fruit and fruit juice) for two weeks. This is important as a gauge to help you determine your relationship with sugar. During the two-week period, stick to just poultry, fish, lean meat, whole-grain products, legumes, nuts, and lots of vegetables, and take note of how you feel. If you run into problems, look over the tips in this section and in the "Nutrient Necessities" section in chapter 9.

12. ▪ **If you complete the two-week elimination diet** and don't notice any adverse symptoms, try adding a naturally sweetened food back into your diet and see how you respond. If the food doesn't bother you, congratulations! Your sugar metabolism is good; you just need to keep it that way. Use this book to learn creative ways to gradually lower your sugar intake without sacrificing taste so you don't run into blood-sugar problems later.

13. ▪ **If you can't complete the elimination diet,** don't feel bad. Most Americans have an unhealthy relationship with sugar because they have overindulged in it for so long. Pay special attention if you notice any of the following scenarios:

14. ▪ **If you experience withdrawal symptoms** such as headaches, moodiness, depression, irritability, and fatigue, you most certainly are addicted to sugar just as others are addicted to coffee or alcohol. Like alcoholics, who need to avoid alcohol, you also need to eliminate all forms of sugar in your diet, at least until your body chemistry improves.

15. ▪ **If you can't go long without eating sugary foods,** you probably have a physical dependence on sugar to give you the quick energy your body is lacking. Switch to eating five or six small, protein-rich meals a day. This will better balance your blood sugar and give you more long-term energy so you're less apt to grab for the sweets.

16. ▪ **If eating sugar seems to make all your symptoms go away magically for a short while,** beware. This is often another sign of sugar addiction. Cut out sugars altogether and reduce the amount of other carbohydrates you eat until your body becomes better balanced.

17. ▪ **If you lose unwanted weight while eliminating sugar,** congratulations! You will experience firsthand what most people don't realize: *Avoiding sugar is the easiest, safest, and most permanent way to stay slim.* It's a plain and simple fact that too much sugar makes you fat. Use the tips in this book to lower your sugar intake for good and stay trim for life.

18. ▪ **If you crave sugar or even complex carbohydrates,** that's almost always a sign that you're not getting enough protein. Emphasize lean meat, poultry, fish, eggs, and properly combined complementary vegetable proteins—and your sugar cravings are likely to diminish.

19. ▪ **If you are a vegetarian,** you might want to consider having your amino acid levels tested. According to medical technologist Don Tyson of Aatron Medical Services in Hawthorne, California, plasma and urine tests reveal that vegetarians are often deficient in the amino acids lysine, methionine, tryptophan, carnitine, and taurine. Without sufficient amounts of these amino acids, vegetarians can develop numerous problems, not the least of which are blood-sugar imbalances and sugar and carbohydrate cravings. If you are interested in receiving more information about the amino acid profile test, see the Aatron Medical Services listing in the resources section.

20. ▪ **When you're under tremendous stress,** the desire for sweets can be intense. It's worth it to hold your desire at bay though. Coping with stress—and maintaining a calm mind and balanced emotions—surprisingly becomes much, much easier when you eat well-balanced, nutritious meals and avoid quick fixes like alcohol, caffeine, and sugar.

21. ▪ **Be sure to get enough sleep and rest.** This is an amazingly simple prescription, but it can play a huge role in helping you overcome the sugar blues. When your body is tired, it wants energy—and that usually translates into sugar binges for quick fixes. If you give your body the rest it needs, you naturally solve your body's energy problem, and its desire for sugar will go away as well.

22. ▪ **Stock healthful, easy-to-grab, sugar-free foods** for sudden cravings when you're overworked, tired, or stressed out. A few good examples are nuts, whole-grain crackers, and low-fat cheese.

23. ▪ **Eat more meals at home** where you can oversee the ingredients. Restaurants are not above adding sugar to the most unlikely foods.

24. ▪ **Keep sweets out of the house.** If they aren't easily available, you'll be less likely to eat them.

25. ▪ **Chew on a cinnamon stick to help you beat your sweet tooth.**

26. ▪ **If and when you do eat sugar,** make sure it's with a well-balanced meal or snack. Eating sugar on an empty stomach can cause an initial high followed by a troublesome sugar low. Once your body experiences this sugar low, it will demand more sugar and this up-and-down sugar cycle will continue.

TOOLS OF THE TRADE

27. ▪ **A blender can help you be a whiz** at whipping up dreamy drinks and desserts with little sugar.

28. ▪ **A food processor is an aide as well** when you're using chopped fresh vegetables and fruits in everything from salads to cookies. The fresher your ingredients, the less you'll miss the sugar.

29. ▪ **A good set of knives will work also.** It's just that the work required to make your heavenly natural concoctions will take a little more time, and muscles.

30. ▪ **A stainless steel steaming rack** doesn't cost a lot but will pay off in health dividends. Use it to make stuffed, steamed fruits for dessert or steamed organic vegetables that are so delicious on their own they don't need a sugary sauce to enhance their flavor.

31. ▪ **Invest in waterless cookware,** the most innovative, amazing cookware that I know of. Without your having to add sugar, salt, fat, or liquid of any kind, food cooks in its own juices at a constant 180 degrees—the temperature that kills off *E. coli, Salmonella,* and other unwanted microorganisms but allows all of the vitamins, minerals, and natural flavors to remain. To cook the tastiest and easiest sugar-free foods you've ever tasted, treat yourself to a Royal Prestige cooking set today. To order or to get more information, call 1-800-888-4353.

32. ▪ **A wide-mouthed thermos is a good purchase** that will come in handy for taking homemade, sugar-free soups, stews, and leftovers wherever you go. Or use it to carry sugar-free hot herbal teas or grain-based coffee substitutes.

33. ▪ **Use measuring spoons and cups to be precise** about the amount of sweeteners you add while cooking. An extra tablespoon of honey might not seem like much, but it adds an extra *18 grams of sugars* to your dish. (That's 72 more calories!)

TASTEFUL TECHNIQUES

34. ▪ **Learn to enjoy the taste of foods as they are** without any added sugar. This may take a little time, particularly if you're currently a sugarholic, but your taste buds will change. If you stick with a low-sugar diet, in time not only won't you like the taste of the sickeningly sweet foods you used to indulge in, but you'll appreciate the subtle but terrific tastes of simply prepared foods.

35. ▪ **Explore the five tastes.** There's more to life than sweetness, you know! In fact, in the ancient five-element theory of food therapy in Chinese medicine, it's taught that too much of one taste can cause imbalance in the body. Most Americans have a love affair with both the sweet taste and the salty taste and don't appreciate the value or experience the pleasure that the other tastes can bring: bitter (as in mustard greens); sour (as in a lemon); and pungent (as in a radish).

36. ▪ **Cut down on salt to lessen your cravings for sugar.** This may sound far-fetched, but it's a tip the Chinese knew about more than five thousand years ago. According to Oriental philosophy, salty foods cause a contraction or tightening of the body's fluids and tissues, while sweet foods do the exact opposite: They cause the body to expand or relax. If you overindulge in salty foods, your body usually craves sweet foods as a way to maintain balance. By cutting down on one, you'll automatically start cutting down on the other. The next time you crave sweets, ask yourself, "Have I been eating too much salt?"

37. ▪ **Our sense of taste is intimately connected with our sense of smell,** a little-mentioned but important piece of information that you can use to increase your enjoyment of subtly sweetened foods. By using fresh aromatic herbs, spices, and natural extracts, your nose will love the smell of the sugar-reduced foods you eat and your taste buds will perceive the foods as sweeter than they really are.

38. ▪ **Develop a fear of commercial desserts,** which not only are sweetened with entirely too much sugar, but also commonly contain white flour, questionable preservatives, and harmful trans-fats (in the form of margarine, shortening, rancid oils, and hydrogenated or partially hydrogenated oils).

39. ▪ **Satisfy your sweet tooth naturally** with fresh fruit or desserts made with natural ingredients. These treats give you vitamins, minerals, and fiber that lifeless desserts made with white flour and white sugar simply don't provide.

40. ▪ **A treat doesn't have to be sweet.** Sometimes it just has to be something new and different, something that breaks up your usual routine. As you begin cutting the sugar out, start exploring interesting, nutritious foods that have recently been rediscovered or become commercially available. This book explores many such foods. Don't be afraid to try them.

SPICING LIFE

41. ▪ **Experiment with spices and herbs,** nature's gifts of flavor to us. Your taste buds might become so intrigued by the flavorful tastes of various herbs and spices such as caraway, sage, and cayenne that you simply no longer need so many sweet tastes to satisfy them.

42. ▪ **Coriander, nutmeg, ginger, and cardamom** are all spices that can make a dish taste sweeter and help satisfy your sweet tooth without adding any sugar.

43. ▪ **Natural vanilla extract and cinnamon are classics** when it comes to upping your perceived level of sweetness. If you don't believe that, try this taste test, passed on to me by cookbook author and health-spa menu consultant Jeanne Jones: Pour a cup of milk and add one teaspoon of vanilla extract and one-quarter teaspoon of cinnamon. Mix thoroughly and ask someone to tell you what you put in it. The answer will almost always be "sugar." Use this common perception to increase your enjoyment of everything from cereal and milk to sugar-free sweet treats.

44. ▪ **Other natural flavoring extracts** open up a world of taste possibilities without any extra sugar. Test your imagination by using flavors such as almond, mint, coconut, or lemon extracts and see how once-boring foods are suddenly transformed into new taste sensations. Look for Spicery Shoppe, Frontier Herbs, and other brands that use natural ingredients in their extracts instead of artificial ones. Artificial colors and flavors are made from such ingredients as coal-tar derivatives and narcotics and definitely don't have a place in a healthy diet.

45. ▪ **Cinnamon, cloves, and bay leaves** might soon be just what the doctor orders to help regulate blood-sugar levels. Test-tube studies conducted at the U.S. Department of Agriculture's Vitamin and Mineral Laboratory have shown that these spices triple insulin's ability to metabolize sugar and remove it from the blood. To give your body extra help maintaining blood sugar balance, add these spices to foods and drinks whenever possible.

46. ▪ **Crush dry herbs and spices with a mortar and pestle** before adding them to a dish. Doing so will release the spices' aroma and dramatically increase the food's flavor.

47. ▪ **Learn the art of infusion** and add a gourmet flair to an everyday oil. Simply soak fresh herbs in a bottle of expeller-pressed oil and season salads or vegetables without any sugar.

THOSE "SUGARLESS" SUGARS

48. ▪ **Giving up sugar is hard,** but don't be tempted to use an artificial sweetener as an alternative. This may seem like an easy way out, but you may be surprised to learn that an artificial sweetener doesn't offer any of its advertised advantages and can cause you plenty of harm, as this section will explain.

49. ▪ **The use of artificial sweeteners hasn't diminished Americans' sugar intake;** it actually seems to have given users more of a sweet tooth! The facts are that since artificial sweeteners became widely used about ten years ago, consumption of sugars has increased by more than 10 percent.

50. ▪ **Artificial sweeteners haven't helped with weight loss either.** In the last decade, Americans have become 30 percent fatter even though the consumption of artificial sweeteners has skyrocketed.

51. ▪ **Aspartame (known as Equal or NutraSweet)** may deplete the body's supplies of chromium, a trace mineral known to play a crucial role in sugar metabolism. Insufficient chromium leads to insulin inefficiency, which, in turn, leads to greater insulin resistance or carbohydrate intolerance.

52. ▪ **NutraSweet, Equal, and Sweet'n Low all are sources of "hidden" sugar.** Believe it or not, even though these sweeteners are advertised as ways to avoid it, sugar—disguised as "dextrose"—is in the ingredients list of each of them.

53. ▪ **The use of aspartame can increase sugar and carbohydrate cravings.** This is because phenylalanine, one of aspartame's components, blocks production of serotonin, a neurotransmitter that sends messages from the pineal gland in the brain. When the body's production of serotonin is out of order, a multitude of symptoms, ranging from premenstrual syndrome to depression, can result. Most important, insufficient serotonin causes more sugar and carbohydrate cravings and increases the likelihood of binge eating.

54. ▪ **More than 75 percent of all nondrug complaints** to the Food and Drug Administration concern aspartame, the Aspartame Consumer Safety Network reports. At least seventy different symptoms and five deaths have been reported to result from its use. In his book *Excitotoxins: The Taste That Kills* (Health Press, 1994), Russell Blaylock, M.D., says that the use of aspartame destroys neurons and is contributing to the development of brain and nervous system disorders such as Alzheimer's disease. If you would like more information about the dangers of aspartame, send a self-addressed, stamped envelope and a $1.00 donation to:

ASPARTAME CONSUMER SAFETY NETWORK
P.O. Box 780634
Dallas, TX 75378

55. ▪ **Using saccharin, another artificial sweetener,** has its own set of risks. Saccharin is a petroleum derivative that is a cocarcinogen, a promoter of other cancer-causing agents in the body. For this reason, it has been banned in foods in such countries as Germany and France for almost a century.

56. ▪ **Mannitol, sorbitol, xylitol, and hydrogenated starch hydrolysate** are also not recommended for use. Classified as sugar alcohols, these noncaloric sweeteners are laxatives and, when taken frequently or in large doses, often cause uncomfortable gastrointestinal bloating, cramps, and diarrhea. Common ingredients in sugar-free chewing gums, sorbitol and mannitol do not promote cavities in the mouth, but they have been shown to nourish and increase the number of *Streptococcus mutans* bacteria that do cause cavities. Even more disturbing are the results of long-term feeding studies involving xylitol, which in large doses was shown to cause tumors and organ injury in animals. Finally, according to Douglas Hunt, M.D., author of *No More Cravings* (Warner Books, 1987), sugar alcohols can stimulate hunger and cause addictive allergies just as sugar can.

57. ▪ **Acesulfame potassium,** commercially sold under the brand name Sunette, is another artificial sweetener that has recently appeared. The Center for Science in the Public Interest has studied the safety issues regarding this sweetener and has concluded that acesulfame potassium probably causes cancer. Add this to the list of sweeteners to avoid.

58. ▪ The best way to kick the sugar habit is to use the suggestions in this book, not to turn to artificial sweeteners, no matter what form they take. The human body simply wasn't designed to deal with these unnatural chemicals. Using them is likely to cause different but equally severe or perhaps more harmful problems than those that sugar causes.

SWEETENERS WORTH NOTING

59. ▪ Dehydrated cane-juice crystals, sold under the commercial name Sucanat, are the easiest sweetening substitute for people who are used to white sugar. Made by evaporating the water from sugarcane juice, Sucanat contains the nutrients that naturally occur in sugarcane. It can be used in the same amount as the sugar required in a recipe, but be careful with it: Most recipes use entirely too much sugar, and even in small amounts, Sucanat can cause adverse symptoms in anyone who is allergic to cane sugar.

60. ▪ Maple syrup is a natural sweetener best used in small amounts. Made from boiled-down maple-tree sap, maple syrup contains a full complement of minerals and is particularly rich in potassium and calcium. Another sweetener, maple sugar, is made when maple syrup is dehydrated. (See tip 88 for additional information.)

61. ▪ Honey is a natural sweetener because it is made by bees, but it is sweeter, has more calories, and raises the blood sugar even more than white sugar. However, truly natural honey has some reported medicinal benefits and contains enzymes and small amounts of minerals, so it does not upset the body's mineral balance as much as refined sugar. In addition, baked goods made with honey have the added benefit of remaining fresher longer than those made with other sweeteners. (See tip 88.)

▪ BONUS TIP: *Never give an infant under eighteen months of age honey or products made with honey. This sweetener sometimes contains trace amounts of botulinum spores, which are easily denatured by the mature digestive tract of an adult but can be harmful or even fatal to an infant, whose digestive tract is just developing.*

62. ▪ **Blackstrap molasses** is the residue after crystals of sugar are removed from beet juice or sugarcane. Although it still contains 65 percent sucrose, blackstrap molasses contains measurable amounts of minerals, especially calcium and iron, making it more nutritious than most other sweeteners. Other types of molasses such as sorghum molasses and Barbados molasses are made from a similar process but are much less nutritious than the blackstrap variety.

63. ▪ **Aguamiel** is a thick, dark, distinctive-tasting sweetener made from maguey cactus plants. With a taste somewhat reminiscent of molasses, aguamiel is best used in small amounts for sweetening bean recipes. If you are interested in trying aguamiel, ask your local health-food store to order it for you.

64. ▪ **Rice amasake, rice syrup, barley malt, and sorghum syrup** are sweeteners prepared by fermenting the grains from which they came. The fermenting bacteria convert the grain starches into simple sugars and also some complex sugars and still retain some complex carbohydrates. In addition, these grain-based liquid sweeteners are at least half-composed of nutrients that are found in the whole grains.

65. ▪ **Rice syrup powder,** sold commercially as Devan-Sweet, is half as sweet as sugar but can be substituted for it in equal amounts to create a less sweet version of a recipe. Made from evaporated rice syrup, it also contains some minerals and complex carbohydrates, as rice syrup does.

66. ▪ **Fruit and dried fruit** are, of course, one of the best ways to sweeten foods. Mashed banana, chopped apple, or a few raisins are just a few ways to naturally satisfy your sweet tooth and get a healthy dose of vitamins and minerals. Just remember, though, that while a little fruit may be healthy, too much fruit can cause all the problems that sugar can cause.

67. ▪ **Date "sugar"** is made from pulverized dried dates. It has the consistency of sugar but isn't refined like sugar. It also contains fiber and is high in many minerals. In addition, since date "sugar" is just dried fruit, it is allowed on sugar-restricted diets. One tablespoon of date "sugar" is counted as one fruit exchange in the diabetic exchange system, a listing of food portions from each food group in which each portion is interchangeable with others in the same group. Look for this sweetener in natural-food stores.

68. ▪ **Fruit juice and fruit juice concentrates,** common ingredients in goodies sold in health food stores, are concentrated sources of sugar that contain the nutrients present in fresh fruit but none of the fiber that balances blood sugar. These sweeteners can quickly flood your bloodstream with sugar, then cause an equally fast fall in blood sugar if they are not balanced with some protein, fat, and fiber. When making your own baked goods or desserts, try to use fruit juice instead of juice concentrates or fruit syrups, which are even more condensed, and be sure to use any juice sweetener judiciously.

▪ BONUS TIP: *Besides giving you all of the sugar from pounds and pounds of fruit, commercial fruit juice and juice concentrates also unfortunately become concentrated sources of the fungicides and pesticides used on all that fruit. For this reason, be sure to go out of your way to buy organic varieties. There's no sense making a goodie full of nutritious ingredients and then ruining it by adding a sweetener full of harmful chemicals.*

69. ▪ **Fructose** is a natural sugar found in fruit that is usually made commercially from corn. A highly refined product, like sugar, it is devoid of nutrients but is included in this book because it scores low (only 20) on the Glycemic Index. In other words, it only stimulates insulin secretion slightly, causing less of a rise and fall in blood-sugar levels and making it tolerated by *some* hypoglycemics and diabetics. Fructose is sweeter than sucrose, so less is needed to obtain the same sweetness in a recipe. As with all sweeteners, use fructose in small amounts if you tolerate it. Large amounts have been shown to increase artery-clogging LDL cholesterol levels, raise uric-acid levels in the blood, and cause diarrhea and gastrointestinal pain in some people. It is also known to raise triglyceride levels more than any other type of sugar. (See tip 87.)

70. ▪ **Stevia** is a sweet herb that is the sweetener of choice for many afflicted with conditions such as *Candida albicans* and parasites. It has been used for hundreds of years as a sweetener in South America and now has wide commercial value in Japan, where it is put in everything from soft drinks to soy sauce. Stevia has thirty times the sweetness of sugar, negligible calories, and does not raise blood sugar like other caloric sweeteners. As of the printing date of this book, the FDA would not allow stevia to be used commercially in foods, but you can still buy the herb from the sources listed in the resources section. Since one teaspoon of white stevia extract powder has the sweetening power of two to four cups of sugar, the most common way to use stevia is to make a liquid concentrate with it (using one teaspoon powder mixed in three tablespoons water) and add a drop or two to sweeten drinks and foods.

71. ▪ **Fructooligosaccharides (FOS)** are sucrose molecules to which one, two, or three additional fructose molecules have been attached. Naturally occurring in some grains and vegetables, FOS provide your taste buds with the taste of sugar, but the molecules are too big to be digested by the body as sugar. Since FOS aren't digested, this sweetener doesn't affect blood-sugar levels. It also can't be utilized by *Candida albicans*, other yeasts, and some bacteria. The best news about FOS, though, is that it provides a benefit that none of the other sweeteners do: It nourishes and promotes the growth of friendly intestinal bacteria such as bifidus and lactobacilli. This makes it a potential good-for-you sweetener for people struggling with yeast infections, parasites, and other gastrointestinal disorders. The Japanese have been using FOS for nearly a decade with no adverse effects reported, though in large doses, it may cause soft stools or diarrhea. FOS is still quite expensive, but it looks as if it could become an important sweetener in the future. If you try it, begin using it sparingly, perhaps one-quarter teaspoon or less at a time to sweeten drinks or cereals.

72. ▪ Determine which natural sweeteners are best for you. One person may feel best using fructose, while another may tolerate honey better. Since our individual body chemistries are so different, the foods we each feel best eating will vary as well.

73. ▪ Use the least concentrated, least sweet, and smallest amounts of sweeteners possible. Remember that a sugar is still sugar to the body, no matter how natural it may be.

SUPERMARKET SAVVY

74. ▪ Concentrate your grocery shopping in the outer aisles. Foods on the inner aisles are designed to have a long shelf life, and sugar is one of the most common preservatives for this purpose. Shop the outer aisles—the produce, meat, dairy, and bulk-foods sections—and take some of the guesswork out of what to buy. It's by far the best way to shop.

75. ▪ **Become a label reader.** There's just no way around it: If you're going to buy packaged foods, you have to pay attention to what's in them. Three-quarters of the sugars Americans ingest are "hidden" in processed foods, so you have to become skeptical about every food you're thinking of buying. Read those labels, educate yourself, and don't let the "hidden" sugar pass by you.

76. ▪ **Label Reading Lesson #1:** Read the number of sugar grams listed on the nutrition-facts label of the food you're considering buying. The lower the number of sugar grams, the better off you are. As a general guideline, look for foods that contain *three grams of sugars or less per serving.*

77. ▪ **If it helps you to understand grams of sugars in terms of teaspoons of sugar,** realize that there are *four grams of sugars in every teaspoon (or packet) of sugar.* A can of soda that has 40 grams of sugar, therefore, is the equivalent of having a can of sparkling water with flavoring, then adding *10 teaspoons of sugar* to it.

78. ▪ **Label Reading Lesson #2:** Compare the number of sugar grams to the number of total carbohydrate grams. Avoid foods that have more than one-third of their total carbohydrates coming from sugars. The majority of the carbohydrates you consume each day should be of the complex variety, not from simple sugars. To help you eat this way, shop for foods with the lowest number of sugar grams in relation to their carbohydrate grams.

79. ▪ **Label Reading Lesson #3:** Peruse the ingredients list and look for sugar in all its various forms. It can be listed as any of the following: barley malt, beet sugar, brown sugar, buttered syrup, cane-juice crystals, cane sugar, caramel, carob syrup, corn syrup, corn syrup solids, date sugar, dextran, dextrose, diastase, diastatic malt, ethyl maltol, fructose, fruit juice and fruit juice concentrate, glucose, glucose solids, golden sugar, golden syrup, grape sugar, high-fructose corn syrup, honey, invert sugar, lactose, malt syrup, maltodextrin, maltose, mannitol, molasses, raw sugar, refiner's syrup, sorbitol, sorghum syrup, sucrose, sugar, turbinado sugar, xylitol, and yellow sugar. These are all ingredients you want to avoid.

80. ▪ **Label Reading Lesson #3 (Short Version):** A quick way to discern sugars on the label is simply to look for the word *sugar* in any form and for words ending in *-ose.*

▪ BONUS TIP: *While you're reading the label for sugar content, pay attention to the other ingredients in the food as well. If there are ingredients that you can't pronounce or spell, much less recognize, the chances are good that the product belongs more in a laboratory experiment than in your body. Skip the fake foods and instead buy products that have identifiable whole foods as ingredients.*

81. ▪ **Label Reading Lesson #4:** Pay attention if a label lists how many fruit exchanges in the diabetic food-exchange system the food counts as. In my experience counseling clients, I have found that even healthy individuals usually do better when they limit themselves to two to four fruit exchanges per day. Even if you aren't diabetic, choose products that count as one fruit exchange or less to avoid overconsumption of even natural sugar-rich, fruit-sweetened foods.

82. ▪ **Understand the meaning of "sugar-free"** under the FDA's new food-labeling rules. It means that the food contains less than 0.5 grams of sugar per serving (a great goal to shoot for).

▪ BONUS TIP: *Be careful of foods with old labels on them or cookbooks that mention they are "sugar-free." Many labels and older cookbooks were printed before the new labeling requirements went into effect, and the foods and recipes in them definitely don't qualify as "sugar-free."*

83. ▪ **"No added sugar," "without added sugar," and "no sugar added"** are recently regulated terms that mean that no sugar or ingredients containing sugars (e.g., fruit juices, applesauce, or dried fruit) were added during the processing or packing of the product, and that the product has no ingredients that were made with added sugars, such as jams, jellies, or concentrated fruit juices.

▪ BONUS TIP: *"Sugar-free" and "no added sugar" signal a reduction in calories from sugars only, not from fat, protein, and other carbohydrates. If the total calories are not reduced, a statement will appear next to the "sugar-free" claim explaining that the food is "not low calorie" or "not for weight control." If the total calories are reduced, the "sugar-free" claim must be accompanied by a "low calorie" or "reduced calorie" claim.*

84. ▪ **A "reduced sugar" product** contains at least 25 percent less sugar than the original product.

85. ▪ **Don't be fooled** by manufacturers looking to capitalize on consumers' desire to buy natural sugars. Although they may sound or look healthier than white sugar, all of the following are fancy terms for refined sugars that give you nothing but empty calories: blond sugar, brown sugar, "natural" sugar, raw sugar, turbinado sugar, and yellow-D sugar.

86. ▪ **While "all natural" is almost always the way to go when it comes to choosing food,** the words *all natural* on a label don't have any real meaning and certainly don't mean that the product is low in sugars. An increasing number of sweeteners—brands such as FruitSource and FruitSweet, for example —are made from all-natural ingredients but are highly concentrated sources of sugars. Use them by the pinch or by the drop if you must, but by all means, do not use them with abandon.

87. ▪ **If fructose is your sweetener of choice,** buy pure crystalline fructose instead of the liquid variety. Liquid fructose is actually isomerized corn syrup.

88. ▪ **Be careful to buy 100 percent pure maple syrup and honey.** If you grab the wrong stuff because it's priced below all the others or because you're in a hurry, you could be buying a mixture of mostly corn syrup instead.

89. ▪ **Don't go grocery shopping when you're hungry.** If your stomach is empty as you browse the aisles, your plummeting blood sugar will tempt you to buy high-sugar items instead of nutritional staples. Eat a well-rounded meal before you go shopping to avoid coming home with bags full of junk food.

THE FINE ART OF MODERATION

90. ▪ **Eat a sweet treat slowly, one small forkful at a time, and savor it.** When you allow yourself to get pure enjoyment from your indulgence, you'll be satisfied with a small amount and won't want to eat the whole thing.

91. ▪ **Better yet, split it.** Your friend or lover will love you for sharing your dessert, and your body will be happier with the arrangement as well.

92. ▪ **Do not restrict yourself to the point of causing a sugar binge.** Human nature is such that we always seem to yearn for the things we can't have. Giving yourself a touch of sweetness here and there may be a better strategy in the long run than total abstinence.

93. ▪ **Try limiting your sugar intake for six days at a time** and then, on the seventh day, allow yourself to eat a serving of any sweet treat you want. This tip helps to instill moderation in those who tend to have an all-or-nothing attitude toward sugar.

94. ▪ **Another moderation strategy is this:** Allow yourself indulgences during vacations or special occasions, but once your regular routine begins again, go back to your low-sugar diet for life. One male friend of mine has made this practice into a real science, being able to maintain his weight despite his occasional culinary "splurges."

95. ▪ **Do the best you can at reducing your sugar intake,** but don't be too hard on yourself. Remember that if you aren't always perfect, it's because you're a human being, not a robot. If you ate more sweets today than you would have liked, accept it and just vow to eat better tomorrow. Mistakes can be helpful if you use them as lessons.

96. ▪ **Avoiding sweets is important for good health,** but just as important is a healthy attitude and a balanced lifestyle. Your desire to cut down on sugar is commendable, but be sure to keep it in perspective with other factors that contribute to a healthy quality of life: avoidance of damaged fats, unnecessary chemicals, and environmental toxins; regular exercise; a positive self-image; and meaningful work and personal relationships.

CHAPTER 2

Get the Sugar Out
of Bed and Breakfast

Most people would never think of trying to start their car in the morning without any fuel or with the wrong type of fuel. They know that the car most likely wouldn't run, or if it did, it certainly wouldn't run efficiently.

But many Americans don't have the same respect for their bodies as they do their cars. They start their day with coffee and a Danish, an instant breakfast shake and a Pop-Tart, or a sugar-laden, fat-free muffin—then wonder why they don't have any energy two hours later. Some even leave the house for a full day of work with nothing in their stomachs at all, yet they are dismayed when they don't experience their optimal level of mental, emotional, and physical functioning later in the day.

Part of getting the sugar out of your diet means you have to treat breakfast as what it really is: the most important meal of the day. Breakfast literally means the break to the fast you experienced since last night's dinner or snack. That's why it's so important. What you have (or don't have) for breakfast can essentially make or break your whole day. Don't be afraid to eat a well-rounded meal in the morning. By doing so, you might just find yourself experiencing more energy than you remembered was possible and getting rid of daily munchies, cravings, and the 10 A.M. sugar blues.

The human body really is an amazing machine. Give it the nutrients it requires and it treats you well. Start it with the right fuel in the morning and it runs efficiently all day long.

The tips in this chapter are designed to help you do just that. They'll teach you how to have a better breakfast that's low in sugar and high in taste.

BREADS AND SPREADS

97. ▪ **Pick out bread that has the lowest amount of sugars per serving.** Don't forget that yeast-raised bread has sugar in it almost by definition. Sugar is added to make yeast multiply and to cause bread to rise. (This phenomenon is a good illustration of why sugar exacerbates yeast problems in those who have *Candida albicans*.)

98. ▪ **Besides just knowing about bread's sugar content,** all sugar-conscious consumers should avoid the bleached flour that most commercial yeasted breads contain. Flour bleach forms alloxan, a compound that has been shown to cause diabetes in animals by destroying the beta cells of the pancreas.

99. ▪ **Whole-grain bread is a taste treat all on its own.** Its texture, flavor, and chewiness beat the blandness of refined white bread hands down. It's so satisfying there's simply no need to top its taste with a sugary jam.

100. ▪ **Sourdough is not only a great change of pace,** it also is a sugar-free and yeast-free way of indulging in bread. Instead of yeast, sourdough bread is naturally leavened with fermenting agents that break down the flour's cellulose structure, neutralize its mineral-inhibiting phytic acid, and release more nutrients into the dough. The result is a more nutritious bread that has no sugar. Look for whole-grain varieties such as those from French Meadow Bakery and Pacific Bakery, which are sold in natural-food stores throughout the country.

101. ▪ **Naturally leavened raisin bread** is a great alternative to a Danish or Pop-Tart for those still weaning themselves from sugar-started mornings. For some, it can even serve as dessert. One client of mine told me she could satisfy her yen for cookies by indulging in a slice of toasted, lightly buttered Kamut Almond-Raisin Bread from Pacific Bakery.

102. ▪ **Sprouted bread is a healthful, sweet way to start your day.** The germination process used to make the bread naturally converts some of the grain's starches to sugars and produces a bread that's so good it's worth a special visit to your local health-food store to buy it. Good brands include Essene Bread from Lifestream Natural Foods or Manna Bread from Nature's Path.

103. ▪ **Toast bread to bring out its sweetness.** If you've got to have a touch of sweetness, this is a great way to do it. Toasting bread converts just enough of its starches to sugars for more sweetness for your taste buds.

104. ▪ **A dab of creamy butter adds a sweet touch** that satisfies many. True, the butter supplies fat, but remember that a little fat is balancing to the blood sugar and improves the ratio of insulin to glucagon, which helps the body access its stored fat for energy.

105. ▪ **For your own cinnamon toast,** sprinkle cinnamon on top of the melted butter. You'll be amazed that this topping has no sugar.

106. ▪ **Yogurt cheese is a delightful spread for bread as well.** To make it, simply line a colander with cheesecloth, place a drip bowl underneath, and put two cups of plain, low-fat yogurt on top of the cheesecloth. Put everything in the refrigerator, let the yogurt drain for several hours or overnight, and what remains is delicious cheese that is a great toast topper.

107. ▪ **Try to get out of the habit of using jam or fruit spread** as a toast topper. An all-fruit spread is a better choice than a sugar-sweetened jam, but only because it uses natural sweeteners instead of refined sugar. Most people are amazed to find out that popular fruit-spread brands such as Polaner All-Fruit and Smucker's Simply Fruit usually contain the *same amount of sugars* as regular sugar-sweetened preserves. That's 8 to 12 grams of sugars in every tablespoon. *Three Sweet Teeth.*

108. ▪ **Low-sugar preserves usually contain about half the amount of sugars** as regular preserves, but they're made with nutrient-depleting refined sugar and artificial colors. It's far better for you to buy an all-fruit spread and dilute it with water for your own low-sugar jam.

109. ▪ **Unsweetened apple butter** is a better choice than jam when you want something sweet. It contains less sugars than preserves—usually 4 to 7 grams per tablespoon—but be sure to use only a tablespoon or less. *Two Sweet Teeth.*

110. ▪ **Another way to get that fruit-sweet flavor with less sugar** is to try Kozlowski Farms brand fruit spreads. Also sweetened with just fruit, Kozlowski Farms spreads have the lowest amount of sugars on the market—*one gram per tablespoon of spread*—and are a boon for anyone who is used to jam but is really serious about lowering his or her sugar intake. Call 707-887-1587 if you have trouble locating these spreads at natural-food stores in your area. *One Sweet Tooth.*

111. ▪ **Or make your own homemade jam.** Just blend and heat the fruit of your choice, add sweet spices if you want, and use as you would any other jam. This is a great way to use up any fruit you have around the house. The variety of possibilities of different fruit spreads that you can make are endless, but here is one example from my administrative assistant, Amy Bondi. *Two Sweet Teeth.*

▪ PEACH BUTTER ▪

2 fresh medium-sized peaches

Peel peaches and slice them into pieces. Add peach pieces to a food processor or blender and whip until smooth. Heat blended peaches on medium-high heat in a saucepan until it boils. Then turn to low and simmer, stirring occasionally, until mixture thickens to desired apple butter–like consistency. *Makes ¼ cup.* ▪

112. ▪ **Or make a veggie butter.** Sweet spreads don't always have to be made with fruit, you know. They can be just as tasty when made with sweet vegetables such as carrots. The following recipe might sound a little strange, but it's a delicious and nutritious alternative to fruit jam. This one comes from *The Good Breakfast Book* by Nikki and David Goldbeck. *One Sweet Tooth.*

▪ CARROT BUTTER ▪

1 cup cooked carrots
2 tablespoons nut butter (see tip 113)
1 teaspoon honey
¼ teaspoon salt (omit if nut butter is salted)

Puree one cup cooked carrots in a food processor or mash with a fork. Beat until smooth with nut butter of your choice, honey, and salt. *Makes ¾ cup.* ▪

113. ▪ **Explore the world of nut and seed butters,** including everything from almond butter to tahini (sesame-seed butter). Peanut butter is always a nutrition-packed favorite, but other butters can offer variety and their own special creaminess to your usual morning toast. Be sure to buy an *unsweetened* nut butter though. Jif and Skippy just won't do it. Look for such brands as Arrowhead Mills, Marantha Natural Foods, or Roaster Fresh by Kettle Foods.

■ BONUS TIP: *See if your local health-food store offers grind-your-own nut butters. Their extrafresh taste can't be beat.*

114. ■ **Melted low-fat cheese** is another way to top your toast—the protein and fat will balance your blood sugar.

BREAKFAST GOODIES

115. ■ **Muffins can be a source of high-quality, balanced nutrition,** but most commercial brands are the furthest thing from this ideal, being sources of empty-calorie sugars and not much more. Be especially careful of fat-free varieties, which often have more sugars than many cookies and cakes.

116. ■ **Check out your local natural-food supermarket,** where you may be able to find homemade, naturally sweetened, but low-sugar goodies that are baked locally.

117. ■ **Or bake your own.** After all, muffins really are quick breads, usually taking not much more than thirty minutes to make from start to finish. If you're unsure of how to use natural sweeteners in your baking, pay special attention to the "Tips for Better Baking" section in chapter 7 and check out some of the fine cookbooks listed in the bibliography.

118. ■ **Use mashed sweet vegetables and fruits**—such as mashed winter squash, bananas, or applesauce—to add natural sweetness and moisture to the muffins you bake. The following recipe, from *Back to Health* by Dennis W. Remington, M.D., and Barbara W. Higa, R.D., uses sweet, creamy pumpkin puree in this way. *One Sweet Tooth.*

▪ WHOLE-GRAIN PUMPKIN MUFFINS ▪

1¼ cups whole-wheat flour
½ cup wheat germ
2½ teaspoons baking powder
½ teaspoon salt
¾ teaspoon ground cinnamon
¾ teaspoon ground nutmeg
2 eggs
2 tablespoons honey
¾ cup milk (or nut milk)
½ cup canned pumpkin puree
¼ cup cold-pressed oil
1 teaspoon natural vanilla extract

Stir together the flour, wheat germ, baking powder, salt, cinnamon, and nutmeg. Make a well in the center. Combine the eggs, honey, milk, pumpkin, oil, and vanilla; add all at once to the dry ingredients. Stir until moistened. Spoon into 12 oiled muffin cups. Bake at 400 degrees for 15–20 minutes. *Makes 12 muffins.* ▪

119. ▪ **Begin easily converting your own favorite muffin recipes** to more nutritious versions by replacing sugar with Sucanat, date "sugar," or brown-rice syrup powder, and by using whole-wheat pastry flour in place of all-purpose flour.

120. ▪ **Use high-protein ingredients** such as nut butters, nuts, seeds, eggs, or "supergrains" such as quinoa, amaranth, or teff to balance out the sugar content of muffins. In this recipe, shared with us by the Arrowhead Mills company, peanut butter adds creamy flavor and moisture—and power-packed nutrition that will keep you going for hours. *Two Sweet Teeth.*

▪ PEANUT BUTTER MUFFINS ▪

2 cups whole-wheat pastry flour
1 tablespoon baking powder
1/2 teaspoon sea salt (optional)
1/4 cup unsweetened, natural-style peanut butter
1/3 cup oil
1/4 cup honey or molasses
1 1/2 cups milk

Stir flour, baking powder, and salt in a bowl. Mix peanut but-
ter, oil, honey, and milk in a separate large bowl until smooth.
Add dry mixture to liquid mixture and mix with minimal
strokes. Do not beat. Fill 12 oiled muffin tins two-thirds full.
Bake in preheated 350-degree oven 25 minutes or until done.
Makes 12 muffins. ▪

121. ▪ **Giving up familiar sweet foods can be difficult,**
but it's not always because it's hard to give up all the sugars in
these foods. Sometimes it's just because we're creatures of habit,
accustomed to foods we grew up with or are used to. Instead of
totally abstaining from traditional favorites, try making low-
sugar versions of foods that are familiar to you. This recipe,
from *Eating for A's* by Alexander Schauss, Barbara Friedlander
Meyer, and Arnold Meyer, is for a healthier version of a Danish
pastry. *Two Sweet Teeth.*

▪ MOCK DANISH PASTRY ▪

2 eggs
1/4 cup low-fat milk or soy milk
2 slices whole-grain bread
cream cheese (or mock cream cheese made from tofu)
    for spreading

juice of ¹⁄₂ lemon
1 teaspoon natural vanilla extract
1 apple and 6 strawberries, chopped,
    or 6 pineapple chunks
2 tablespoons raisins
¹⁄₂ teaspoon ground cinnamon

Preheat oven to 400 degrees. Beat eggs and milk together and saturate bread, as for French toast. Lightly grease a baking pan and bake bread slices for 5 minutes, then remove from oven. Whip cream cheese, lemon juice, and vanilla together. Spread on each slice of bread. Mix fruit and raisins; place on top of each slice of bread. Gently roll up slice, securing with a toothpick. Sprinkle cinnamon on top and bake for another 3 minutes. Serve warm as is or cut into small pieces. *Makes 4 pastries.* ▪

PANCAKE PARADISE

122. ▪ **Don't give up pancakes** just because you have to give up white flour and white sugar. Try whole-grain varieties instead and you'll never again want to go back to those made with all-purpose flour. Two convenience products that can help you enjoy with little fuss the delightful, light, almost nutty flavor of whole-grain pancakes are Arrowhead Mills' Multi-Grain Pancake Mix and Bob's Red Mill 10-Grain Mix. Look for them by name.

123. ▪ **Take any basic pancake recipe** and put your own stamp on it. By using different herbs, spices, fruit, flavoring extracts, and unrefined oils, you can literally make the pancakes differently every time you make them, depending upon your mood, and you'll be adding flavor without refined sugar. The only thing stopping your culinary creations is the inhibition of your imagination. Here are a few ideas to get you started:

124. ▪ **Add ¼ teaspoon pumpkin pie spice** to the pancakes and have your own Thanksgiving.

125. ▪ **Make the cakes maple-y.** Include some natural maple flavoring and a teaspoon or two of maple syrup for a whole new flavor. *One Sweet Tooth.*

126. ▪ **Add some fresh blueberries to the pancake batter.** Practically no one can resist fresh blueberry pancakes right off the griddle. *One Sweet Tooth.*

127. ▪ **Simply add a few drops of vanilla for a sweeter taste.**

128. ▪ **Go nutty.** If you're nuts about almonds, use expeller-pressed almond oil in the recipe and a dash of almond extract. Top with almond butter or home-toasted sliced almonds for pure almond joy. Get the idea? Now let your creativity guide you. . . .

129. ▪ **Baby food isn't just for babies.** It also happens to be a special secret ingredient in many successful sugar-free sensations. (Shh! Don't tell anyone. Word might get around.) If you're on the run and don't have time to spend all morning in the kitchen, try "babying" yourself with the luxury of these little helpers, as nutritionist Melissa Diane Smith has done in this recipe. Brown-rice flour is used here to allow the special sweetness of the sweet potato to shine through. *One Sweet Tooth.*

▪ MELISSA'S SWEET POTATO PANCAKES ▪

1 egg (or 1½ teaspoons Ener-G Egg Replacer
    mixed in 2 tablespoons water)
1 4-ounce jar Earth's Best Sweet Potato baby food

1½ tablespoons expeller-pressed oil
½ a baby-food jar full of water (or ¼ cup)
¾ cup brown-rice flour

Preheat nonstick skillet on medium temperature. Begin by whipping the egg with a fork or making the egg replacer. Add the sweet-potato baby food and the oil. Instead of measuring the water in a measuring cup, add water to the emptied baby-food jar until the jar is half-full. Then put lid on top of the jar, shake it a couple of times, and empty its contents into the liquid ingredients. (This helps you get all of the baby food out of the jar.) Mix all the liquid ingredients together, add the brown-rice flour, and mix again. Drop batter into thin, 2-inch-round, silver-dollar pancakes and cook until brown on one side. Flip over, push the pancakes down, and cook until done. *Serves 2 to 3 people.* ▪

Note: If you want the pancakes to taste more nutty instead of creamy, add ¼ cup finely chopped pecans to the batter right before cooking.

130. ▪ **Say good-bye to Aunt Jemima pancake syrup (and others like it).** The first three ingredients in the original syrup are corn syrup, sugar syrup, and high-fructose corn syrup—all refined sweeteners that are nutrient-depleted as well as nutrient-depleting.

131. ▪ **Reach for 100 percent pure maple syrup** if you must top your pancakes with something sweet. Sure, maple syrup is high in natural sugars, but it also contains nutrients that the imitation syrups just don't have. In addition, it has a distinctive, robust taste that can't be beat. Maple syrup is very concentrated though—*a tablespoon contains 13 grams of sugars*—so get into the habit of dabbing it on pancakes one drop at a time.

132. ▪ **Or use maple syrup diluted with water or almond milk.** Pure maple syrup is so concentrated that most people will want less on their pancakes if they taste their food before they pour the syrup on. But if you always pour on more than you need, dilute the syrup first.

133. ▪ **Unsweetened applesauce also tops pancakes well,** but try not to use more than one-half cup (which is one fruit exchange) on your stack of cakes. For a sweet change of pace, explore the different varieties of unsweetened fruit applesauces —such as strawberry applesauce or peach applesauce from Solana Gold or Santa Cruz Natural.

134. ▪ **Try to use fruit instead of syrups and spreads on pancakes.** Whether chopped, sliced, whole, or blended, fruit is nature's most perfect sweetener.

BREAKFAST ENTRÉES

135. ▪ **Have a substantial breakfast that includes ade-quate protein and fiber** if you have blood-sugar problems. If high-sugar foods make up your meal, you're apt to spend the rest of the day with erratic blood-sugar levels, not feeling well and prone to going into munchie mayhem.

136. ▪ **Enjoy some eggs-ceptional breakfasts** with eggs, of course. They are a nearly perfect food that has gotten an unfair rap from the media and some health professionals recently. While eggs do contain cholesterol, dietary cholesterol only becomes a problem when it becomes altered because of smoking, curing, or aging processes, as in such foods as sausage, aged cheese, and meats. Enjoy eggs in moderation and use them as great sources of protein to balance blood sugar quickly.

137. ▪ **Another reason to eat eggs** is that they may very well help blood-sugar metabolism. You see, each insulin molecule that works to balance blood sugar contains eight atoms of sulfur, a trace mineral that eggs supply in abundance. Many antidiabetic drugs also contain sulphur, so it's reasonable to assume that eating sulfur-rich foods such as eggs can help your insulin work more effectively.

138. ▪ **Tired of eggs and toast?** For an exotic twist to your usual morning meal, try it the Oriental way. Fry up leftover brown rice and a scrambled egg in two teaspoons of canola or sesame oil. Top with green onion tops and a bit of parsley if you like or a dash of dark sesame oil. This dish gives you complex carbohydrates, protein, and healthy fat—everything you need to begin your day the balanced blood-sugar way!

139. ▪ **Skip the ham or bacon.** Although they contain protein, they also contain entirely too much sugar as well as saturated fat, altered (or oxidized) cholesterol, and potentially carcinogenic chemicals.

140. ▪ **To replace high-sugar sausage** (which is also high in fat and salt), make your own. Use lean ground turkey or ground beef and add flavorful herbs such as garlic and fennel. Here's an example shared with me by nutritionist Melissa Diane Smith:

▪ HOMEMADE TURKEY SAUSAGE ▪

1 pound lean ground turkey (Shelton's brand preferred)
2–6 garlic cloves, crushed and pressed
$\frac{1}{2}$ teaspoon rubbed sage
$\frac{1}{2}$ teaspoon ground fennel

Preheat oven to 350 degrees. Mix the above ingredients, shape the meat mixture into 2-inch-round sausage patties, and place on a broiler pan or on a wire rack above a baking pan. Bake until done and no pink remains in the center, about 20–25 minutes. Add sea salt to taste at the table if necessary. *Serve 3 to 4 people.* ▪

141. ▪ Expand your breakfast repertoire. Break through the bonds of traditional breakfast foods. Your morning meal doesn't have to consist of eggs, sausage, toast, or cereal. It can be anything that's low in sugar and that gets you off to a good start. Leftovers from last night's dinner work well in a pinch.

142. ▪ Cooked chicken, turkey, or lean beef can fill your protein bill when you have no eggs left in the fridge.

143. ▪ Or try low-fat cottage cheese. (If you don't like it plain, try adding cinnamon on top for a sweeter taste.)

CEREALS AND MILKS TO TOP THEM

144. ▪ Cereals are one of the top places you need to watch out for sugars. Hidden in some of the healthiest-looking cereals are sugars in every disguised form imaginable. Review the list of sugar names in tip 79 before you shop for cereals and be sure to pick out a whole-grain brand with *three grams of sugars or less per serving,* if at all possible.

145. ▪ Stick with basics like unsweetened shredded wheat and unsweetened oatmeal. They may not be fancy but they offer wholesome, sugar-free nutrition.

146. ▪ Cream of wheat and cream of rice are also good choices but make sure to buy the whole-grain varieties (such as Arrowhead Mills' Bear Mush and Rice N Shine, Bob's Red Mill Creamy Wheat and Creamy Rice Cereals, or Lundberg Farms Rice Cereal). Popular commercial brands of these cereals that are made from refined carbohydrates lack fiber and many nutrients found in the original grain and raise the blood sugar quickly.

147. ▪ If you grab sugar-rich, ready-to-eat cereals because you simply don't have time to make hot whole-grain cereals in the morning, then make them the night before—in the oven, that is! There's nothing nicer than waking up to the smell of cooked whole-grain cereal that's ready for you to eat. Here is an overnight recipe for cooking cereal grains that I learned from my 106-year-old mentor, Dr. Hazel Parcells.

▪ OVERNIGHT WHOLE-GRAIN CEREAL ▪

$2\frac{1}{2}$ cups water, boiling
1 cup grains (rolled oats, cornmeal, cracked wheat,
    barley grits, or brown rice)
1 teaspoon salt

Using a casserole pot, pour the $2\frac{1}{2}$ cups boiling water over the grains and add the salt. Preheat oven to 350 degrees. Place casserole in oven, reducing heat to 200 degrees. The cereal will cook in about two hours, or it may remain in the oven all day or all night without reducing the nutritional values. To make larger quantities, use the same proportions of liquids to dry materials. *Serves 4.* ▪

148. ▪ **Use natural liquid sweeteners sparingly,** by the drop, on your cereals. A little molasses, honey, or maple syrup can go a long, long way.

149. ▪ **Better yet, use fruit as a natural cereal sweetener.** A few sliced peaches, strawberries, or blueberries can brighten your bowl.

150. ▪ **Granola may seem like a health food,** but its sugar content often puts it in the same league as many desserts. Pick the brand you buy carefully or make your own so you can control its sugar content. Try the following recipe, which appeared in *The Yeast Connection Cookbook* by William Crook, M.D., and Marjorie Hurt Jones, R.N. It is the lowest-sugar granola I have ever seen, but it is still absolutely delicious. *One Sweet Tooth.*

▪ OAT GRANOLA ▪

3 cups rolled oats
$\frac{1}{2}$ cup sunflower seeds
$\frac{1}{2}$ cup almonds, halved or coarsely chopped
1–2 teaspoons ground cinnamon
$\frac{1}{4}$ teaspoon salt (optional)
$\frac{1}{4}$ cup oil
$\frac{1}{4}$ cup pineapple juice
$\frac{1}{2}$ cup mashed banana

Preheat oven to 350 degrees. Combine oats, seeds, almonds, cinnamon, and salt in a large mixing bowl. In a blender jar, combine the oil, pineapple juice, and mashed banana, and blend briefly. Pour the thick liquid over the oat mixture and blend well. Spread on a large jelly-roll pan (cookie sheet with edges) and bake for about 40–45 minutes, stirring the granola 2 or 3 times. When lightly brown, remove from the oven—it crisps as it cools. Store the cooled granola in tightly capped glass jars, in a cool place. *Makes about 6 cups.* ▪

151. ▪ **Toss together your own muesli** and eliminate altogether the honey, maple syrup, and fruit juice used to sweeten granola. A muesli really is a hodgepodge, and it can be as individualistic as you are. Common muesli ingredients to include in any way you see fit are uncooked rolled oats; corn or wheat flakes; unsweetened puffed cereals such as puffed rice; seeds and chopped nuts; and chopped fruit such as apples or dried fruit such as raisins or dates.

152. ▪ **Milk may seem like a natural,** but remember it's naturally high in milk sugars. In one cup of milk, there's *11 grams of sugars,* so go easy using it on your cereal.

153. ▪ **Lactose-reduced milk** can help eliminate the unwanted bloating and digestive upset milk can cause in most of the world's population. Unfortunately, though, the sugars in this product are even more rapidly absorbed than the sugars naturally present in milk and can cause blood-sugar problems. Diabetics especially need beware.

154. ▪ **Almond milk, soy milk, and rice milk** are helpful for people who have trouble digesting cow's milk, and they can substitute for milk as cereal toppers and recipe ingredients. But keep in mind that they mostly consist of sugars, just like milk. Using any type of sugar-rich milk on a sweet cereal can send your blood sugar soaring (and then falling), so use all milks judiciously.

▪ BONUS TIP: *You can make sugar-free almond milk at home by blending raw or soaked almonds (or a commercial product called Ener-G Nut-Quik) with water.*

BREAKFAST BEVERAGES

155. ▪ **The best drink to begin your day** is pure, filtered water. It's the perfect sugar-free antidote for your thirst and for your body, which has been without it all night long.

156. ▪ **Just say no to juice as a breakfast beverage.** Although it may seem like the ultimate in a healthy drink, whether it's from a container or straight from your juicer, juice is one of the quickest ways to give your pancreas a shock and throw your blood sugar so off-kilter that you might feel out of balance all day long. In one eight-ounce glass of apple juice, for example, you get all of the natural sugars from the three and a half pounds of apples used to make the juice and none of the blood-sugar-balancing fiber. If you start your morning this way, you may experience an initial high, but you're sure to suffer from an eventual blood-sugar low that will leave you wanting more sugar.

157. ▪ **If you can't give up juice just yet,** gradually begin diluting fruit or vegetable juice with more and more water to wean yourself away from the high-sugar content of straight juice. In time, you'll find that a little juice goes very far.

158. ▪ **Use herbal tea** as another, more interesting way to thin out juice. One client of mine begins her day with iced Red Zinger and a little bit of cherry juice, while another goes for mint tea with a touch of apple juice. The choices really are endless. Be creative and see what tasty drink concoctions you can devise to lessen your juice intake.

159. ▪ **If you think you're doing well to gulp down an instant breakfast drink in the morning,** think again. No matter how many nutrients a drink mix such as Carnation Instant Breakfast Drink may contain, it doesn't do you much good when there are *22 grams of sugars* per serving. It's better for you to make a shake such as this one from *Healing with Whole Foods* by Paul Pitchford and swallow a good, sugar-free multivitamin. *Two Sweet Teeth.*

▪ ALMOND MILK SHAKE ▪

¼ cup almonds (soaked, as described below)
2 cups warm water
Dash of sea salt
½ cup fresh fruit *or* 2 tablespoons grain coffee
    or ½ cup carob powder

Soak nuts in water overnight. Drain and discard soaking water. Blend (in a blender) all the ingredients together and serve. *Serves 2.* ▪

160. ▪ **If you're looking for one more reason to convince yourself to give up coffee,** this may be it: Coffee is bad for your blood sugar. It provides a temporary lift but taxes your pancreas and adrenals, which in turn control your blood-sugar-balancing mechanisms. It also causes blood-sugar-balancing minerals to be washed out of your system. Chalk up these reasons and you might just have enough incentive to give up coffee for good.

161. ▪ **Coffee with sugar is double trouble.** Not only does the sugar stimulate the pancreas into activity, but the caffeine prompts the adrenals to induce the liver to convert its stored energy into even more sugar in the bloodstream. Essentially, it's a sugar double whammy! If you feel you must drink coffee, give your pancreas a break: Cut down on the amount you drink, switch to the water-processed decaffeinated variety, and learn to drink it without sweetening.

▪ BONUS TIP: *Coffee substitutes made out of such ingredients as chicory and dandelion roots are tasty ways to help satisfy the desire for a coffeelike taste without the caffeine of coffee.*

162. ▪ **Flavored coffees are quite the rage these days,** but guess what most of them are flavored with? Sugar, of course— that nasty five-letter word. In place of sugar, try adding natural flavoring extracts to decaf coffee and coffee substitutes to give them that gourmet flair. Here's one tasty example:

▪ FRENCH VANILLA CAFÉ ▪

Hot water
1 bag roasted dandelion root or chicory tea
    (or 1 heaping teaspoon Caffix or other grain-based
    coffee substitute)
$1/2$ teaspoon natural vanilla extract

Boil water in a teakettle. Pour boiling water over dandelion or chicory tea bag in coffee cup and let it steep for 5–10 minutes (or over instant grain-based coffee substitute and stir). Add $1/2$ teaspoon vanilla extract, stir, and enjoy. *Serves 1.* ▪

171. ▪ **Be cautious when buying fat-free soups.** Remember, fat-free doesn't necessarily mean sugar-free. Instead, it often means that ingredients such as sugar, corn syrup, honey, and fruit juice have replaced the fat.

172. ▪ **Whole-wheat, oat, brown-rice, or chickpea flour** can thicken a cream soup just as nicely as all-purpose flour—and more nutritiously.

173. ▪ **Sweet starchy vegetables such as squash can thicken cream soup** or even make a creamlike soup all by themselves. Here's a simple, slightly sweet, and utterly creamy recipe I came up with for my book *Super Nutrition for Menopause:*

▪ **BUTTERNUT BISQUE** ▪

4 cups water
1 large butternut squash, skinned and cubed
½ teaspoon salt (optional)
¼ teaspoon ground cumin
¼ teaspoon ground coriander
¼ teaspoon fresh-grated ginger
¼ teaspoon garlic powder
4 sprigs fresh parsley for garnish
12 toasted almonds for garnish
6 tablespoons nonfat yogurt

Place water and squash in soup pot. Cover and simmer for 5 minutes. Add salt, cumin, coriander, ginger, and garlic. Continue simmering for 15 minutes. Serve garnished with a sprig of parsley, chopped toasted almonds, and a dollop of yogurt. *Serves 6.* ▪

▪ ▪ ▪

SALAD DAYS

174. ▪ **Salads are naturally low in sugar and good for your blood sugar.** When they're chock-full of dark green leafy lettuce and vegetables ranging from artichoke hearts to zucchini, salads are loaded with vitamins and minerals that your body needs to maintain optimal blood-sugar levels.

▪ BONUS TIP: *Judge the nutrition of your salad by the richness of its color. Pale iceberg lettuce is much lower in minerals than its darker green cousins and, therefore, not as helpful for your blood sugar. If you're used to iceberg lettuce, try adding a few darker green lettuce leaves (such as red or green loose-leaf or romaine) to your regular salad to increase its nutritional content.*

175. ▪ **Buy the freshest ingredients possible** so your salad is flavorful all on its own. When your vegetables are crunchy and tasty, you'll want to taste more of them and less of a sugar-containing dressing.

176. ▪ **Add some interest to your salad** by including some vegetables you haven't tried before. Any vegetable you would add to salad is essentially sugar-free, so feel free to experiment.

177. ▪ **If you're looking for some sweetness in your bowl of greens,** try using grated carrots or beets. Both are amazingly sweet and add vibrant color to your salad as well. *One Sweet Tooth.*

178. ▪ **As an herb or as a vegetable,** fennel brings its subtly sweet, licoricelike flavor to any food it accompanies. For a change of pace in your salad, try adding sliced strips of fresh fennel.

179. ▪ **Have you ever tried jicama?** If not, you're missing a real treat. Naturally sweet, crisp, and mild, jicama is a tuberlike vegetable that is eaten raw and is a special addition to salads for many people. Try it the next time you get an opportunity.

180. ▪ **Croutons and bacon bits are the only weak links** in the otherwise sugar-free typical salad fare. Hiding in these salad toppers are sugar and high-fructose corn syrup. If you really want croutons, make them at home by adding herbs and garlic to whole-grain bread cubes and oven-toasting them, but skip the bacon bits altogether.

181. ▪ **Adding leftover strips of chicken or turkey or flaked tuna** to a salad can make a satisfying, sugar-free meal-in-one that's especially nice for lunch on a hot summer day.

182. ▪ **Pasta salad is a light meal—light on nutrition, that is.** Believe it or not, the refined pasta found in most commercial salads is, nutritionally, almost in the same category as sugar: It supplies calories but few nutrients. To increase the mineral and fiber content of this meal and to help your blood sugar, be sure to use whole-grain pasta.

183. ▪ **You can also take your favorite pasta salad recipe** and use leftover whole grains in place of the pasta. Brown rice, bulgur wheat, barley, and quinoa all work well in pasta-salad recipes.

DRESSED FOR SUCCESS

184. ▪ **A salad dressing is one place sugar grams can pile up quickly** if you don't choose the dressing you use with care. Watch out for hidden sugars in all dressings, but especially try to avoid fat-free ones made with fruit juices or honey.

185. ▪ **If you're used to honey-based dressings,** wean yourself away from commercial brands that have additional sugars in them and start yourself off with a naturally sweet homemade dressing such as this tasty one from *The Allergy Self-Help Cookbook* by Marjorie Hurt Jones, R.N. *Two Sweet Teeth.*

▪ SESAME-LIME SALAD DRESSING ▪

⅓ cup sunflower oil
3 tablespoons lime juice
2 tablespoons chopped onion
1 tablespoon honey
2 teaspoons sesame seeds
2 mint leaves (optional)

Place the oil, lime juice, onion, honey, sesame seeds, and mint leaves in a blender. Process until smooth. *Makes ⅔ cup.* ▪

186. ▪ **Gradually thin out sweet dressings,** such as the one above, with water as your taste and desire for sweets lessen. *One Sweet Tooth.*

187. ▪ **Vinegar-and-oil dressing is a tried-but-true dressing.** Simple and delicious, it's one of the best ways to stay away from hidden sugars in your dressing.

▪ BONUS TIP: *There are a lot of vinegars from which to choose, and each one gives its own unique flavor. Some nice ones to try are balsamic vinegar, red-wine vinegar, and rice vinegar.*

188. ▪ **Make an herb vinegar** for an extraspecial dressing ingredient. To make it, fill a glass bottle or jar with approximately one cup of fresh herbs such as dill, thyme, rosemary, or tarragon. Add one quart of cider vinegar, red-wine vinegar, or white vinegar, cap the bottle and label it, and let it stand in a cool, dark place. After three to four weeks, it's ready to use.

189. ▪ **Avoid fruit-flavored vinegars such as raspberry or blueberry vinegar.** Both fruit and refined sugar are used to flavor these trendy salad toppers.

190. ▪ **The sweetness and sourness of lemon or lime juices** are naturals in salad dressings. Combine them with olive oil and crushed garlic or herbs if you wish to make a healthy dressing to season your salad.

191. ▪ **If you want a bit more pizzazz added to lemon and oil,** try using sugar-free mustard as I did in this easy-to-make dressing from my first book, *Beyond Pritikin:*

▪ FRENCH OLIVE OIL DRESSING ▪

$1/2$ cup extra-virgin olive oil
2 tablespoons fresh lemon juice
1 teaspoon Dijon mustard
$1/4$ teaspoon salt (optional)

Put all the ingredients in a small, covered jar. Shake vigorously for 30 seconds and refrigerate. Remove from the refrigerator at least an hour before serving to liquefy the oil. *Makes $1/2$ cup.* ▪

192. ▪ **Transform your oil into a salad dressing all by itself** through the art of herbal infusion. Follow tip 47. Olive oil makes a particularly good herbed oil.

193. ▪ **Or transform your oil by vigorously shaking it with tasty herbs.** Here's an example: In a small, covered jar, put $1/2$ cup sesame or peanut oil, $11/2$ tablespoons finely chopped ginger, 1 tablespoon chopped parsley, and 1 minced clove of garlic. Shake the ingredients well and pour on top of your salad.

194. ▪ **Salsa by itself or combined with canola oil makes a quick, terrific dressing** that gives a definite kick to your salad greens.

195. ▪ **A nice change of pace is an avocado-based dressing.** Full of flavor without any sugar, this dressing is from *Cooking for Healthy Healing* by Linda Rector-Page:

▪ ▪ ▪

▪ CALIFORNIA GUACAMOLE DRESSING ▪

1 sliced avocado
$\frac{1}{2}$ sliced red onion
juice of $\frac{1}{2}$ lemon
$\frac{1}{4}$ cup light salsa
3 tablespoons oil (I personally use avocado oil)
2 tablespoons cider vinegar
$\frac{1}{2}$ teaspoon lemon pepper
1 tomato

Blend all the ingredients in a blender until smooth. Pour into a bowl and chop in the tomato. *Makes 1½ cups.* ▪

196. ▪ **Greek Tszitziki Sauce,** a cooling combination of cucumber, herbs, and unsweetened yogurt, can make a refreshingly different salad dressing either by itself or mixed with water, oil, or lemon juice. *It's simple to prepare, too.*

▪ GREEK TSZITZIKI SAUCE ▪

$\frac{1}{3}$ cucumber, peeled, seeded, and diced
1 cup plain, low-fat yogurt
1 clove garlic, minced, *or* 1 green onion, chopped
1 tablespoon fresh dill weed *or* 1½ teaspoons dried dill
    weed *or* 1 tablespoon fresh mint *or* 1½ teaspoons
    dried mint

Combine all the ingredients in a bowl, cover, and chill for a few hours. *Makes 1 cup.* ▪

197. ▪ **If you're used to making a dressing from a mix,** did you know that sugar is a component of almost all of those handy mixes? One exception is The Spice Hunter, which makes a complete line of mixes that are both salt- and sugar-free.

198. ▪ **Two good bottled salad-dressing lines to try** are Cardini's and Paula's, both of which are found in natural-food stores. Both lines contain no sugar and have several delicious varieties from which to choose. (Don't choose Paula's No-Oil Dressings, though. Like many fat-free dressings, these *do* contain sugar.)

CHAPTER 4

Get the Sugar Out
of Entrées and Side Dishes

Getting the sugar out of entrées and side dishes involves a shift in thinking. Instead of worrying about every drop of even naturally occurring fat in the foods you serve, your focus should turn to eliminating processed convenience foods that contain refined carbohydrates and hidden sugars. Doing so will not only help get the sugar out of your diet, but it will also help get the fats you should avoid out of your diet as well. (Packaged foods that contain hidden sugars often contain harmful trans-fats such as hydrogenated oils as well.)

If you stop to think about it, our ancestors survived very nicely eating whatever animal products and plant foods they could find. What they didn't eat was a continual supply of hidden sugar—and this is where Americans have gotten into trouble.

No one wants to spend all day cooking in the kitchen, but when TV dinners and mixes such as Hamburger Helper make up your meals, sugar becomes one of the biggest components of your diet. So what are you to do?

If, like most people, you value convenience above all else, the answer is to find smart ways of enjoying convenience without all that sugar. One way to do that is to plan ahead and make your own convenience foods. Roasting a turkey breast on Sunday afternoon doesn't take a lot of effort, but it can give you ready-to-use, sugar-free turkey meat that will be a godsend later on in the week for making quick sandwiches and such dishes as turkey tetrazzini or turkey hash. Making extra portions of such dishes as lasagna and stir-fries doesn't take much more work, but it can give you a way to enjoy heat-and-serve complete meals when you come home from work and are just too tired to cook.

Another way of coping is to seek out brands of products that give you equal convenience but far superior nutrition than the commercial brands. Finding these products sometimes means making a visit to your local natural-food store, but the rewards you receive (less sugar, more nutrition, better taste, and convenience) make it well worth the trip.

Unlike other diet plans that you might have followed, getting the sugar out of the entrées and side dishes you eat does not in the slightest involve deprivation. In fact, it means experiencing more pure pleasure by eating delicious, fresher-tasting lunches and dinners than before. You can eat "real food" again —food that is wholesome, satisfying, and truly energizing. And you can enjoy dinners as varied as a broiled steak, baked potato, and a salad, to a chicken-and-vegetable stir-fry, to black beans and brown rice.

Getting the sugar out of entrées and side dishes is not that difficult or mysterious, really. The more you stick with unprocessed natural foods (such as the ones recommended in this chapter), the less of a problem sugar will be.

■ ■ ■

MEATY MATTERS

199. ▪ **Meat has received so much bad press in the last decade** that many people are afraid to eat even small amounts. That's unfortunate because, as I explain in my book *Your Body Knows Best*, some people just can't thrive without it. Sure, meat contains some naturally occurring fat, but our bodies are designed to deal with some fat. It's sugar that's the real troublemaker.

200. ▪ **Stick with unprocessed meat** that is baked, broiled, or stir-sautéed. Meat starts to cause problems with your health when it is highly processed —fried, smoked, cured, or aged and loaded with salt and sugar. Avoid meat products with concealed sugar—hot dogs, sausage, ham, and luncheon meats such as bologna and pastrami.

▪ BONUS TIP: *The antibiotics and hormones used to produce most meat these days pose potential problems for your health. Whenever possible, buy organically raised meats that are free of these harmful chemicals. Some poultry brands that offer organically raised chickens and turkeys are Shelton Farms, Harmony Farms, Foster Farms, and Young's Farm. Brands of beef to look for include Country B3R Meats and Coleman Natural Meats.*

201. ▪ **Go ahead and have a lean cut of steak.** It's the steak sauce you should be more concerned about. Some steak sauces have up to *eight grams of sugars per tablespoon*. If you use two tablespoons, that's the sugar equivalent of putting a half-cup serving of chocolate pudding on your steak!

202. ▪ **Eating lean red meat and poultry** is one of the best ways to perk up malfunctioning adrenal glands, an increasingly common problem among people who are overstressed and overworked. This is important because the adrenal glands are intimately involved in sugar metabolism. By eating such foods as lean meats, which help your adrenals function better, you help stabilize your blood-sugar levels.

203. ▪ **Beef, pork, lamb, chicken, and turkey** are all significant sources of zinc, a mineral that is crucial to proper blood-sugar functioning but one that is deficient in more than 60 percent of the American population. (Beef and lamb, the meats people have been avoiding the most recently, are the two highest sources.) Not only is zinc an essential mineral for optimal adrenal function, but it also helps the beta cells of the pancreas both store and release insulin as required. Pancreatic tissues of diabetics have been shown to have one-third the zinc of those of nondiabetics. Do your pancreas a favor and don't hesitate to eat small but frequent portions of these zinc-rich, sugar-free foods.

▪ BONUS TIP: *Whether you eat more lean poultry or heavier red meats should depend a lot on your metabolism. My book* Your Body Knows Best *goes into this in great detail, but generally, individuals who have slow metabolisms feel much better eating such lean animal products as white-meat chicken and turkey, while people with fast metabolisms tend to thrive on higher-fat lamb and beef.*

204. ▪ **If the idea of eating meat is hard for you to swallow,** consider this: Eating meat causes your body to release glucagon, the hormone that works in direct opposition to insulin and helps your body burn off fat stores. Eating "lighter fare" such as pasta, potatoes, and bread causes the pancreas to release more insulin, which can lead to erratic blood-sugar highs and lows and, in many people, can really add on the pounds. While too much meat in the diet can be bad for your health, too little meat can be just as harmful. Two three-ounce portions per day is a good amount for most people. (As an easy guide, a three-ounce portion is the size of a deck of cards.)

205. ▪ **Don't skip eating meat to make room for dessert.**

Although this plan sounds as if it would work calorie-wise, it's likely to backfire on you. You see, eating lean meat is one of the best ways to meet your daily protein requirements. Without adequate protein to help stabilize your blood-sugar and energy levels, your body will crave and you will probably overeat high-carbohydrate foods such as sugar-rich desserts to give you the quick energy you are lacking.

206. ▪ **Combine just a small amount of lean meat** (three ounces or so) with lots of vegetables (as you do in stir-fries and fajitas) to create a naturally balanced meal that's both low in sugars and stabilizing for your blood sugar.

207. ▪ **Tacos can be a low-sugar, balanced meal** as long as you avoid commercial taco-seasoning mixes that contain sugar. One brand that doesn't contain sugar is Hain Taco Seasoning Mix. Instead of a mix you can use a teaspoon of chili powder and half a teaspoon of onion powder to season one pound of ground meat.

208. ▪ **If you shake, then bake, your chicken,** you might be surprised to learn that bleached flour and four types of sugars are listed in the original Shake 'n Bake recipe mix. Here's a way to "quick-coat and bake" your chicken without all that sugar:

▪ QUICK-COAT CHICKEN DRUMSTICKS* ▪

6 chicken drumsticks (or thighs)
½ cup chicken stock (without sugar)
¼ teaspoon canola oil
1 cup crushed shredded wheat
¼ teaspoon garlic powder
¼ teaspoon onion powder
¼ teaspoon dried parsley leaves

*This recipe was adapted from a recipe for Presto Crunchy Drumsticks in *Smart Chicken* by Jane Kinderlehrer.

Wash and skin chicken. Combine chicken stock and oil in a small bowl. In another bowl, mix together the shredded wheat and herbs. Preheat oven to 350 degrees. Dip the chicken in the stock-oil combination, then roll in the coating mixture. Bake until golden brown on the outside, about 45–55 minutes. *Serves 3.* ▪

Note: If you prefer a finer coating, you can blend the shredded wheat in a blender until fine, like a flour, before coating.

209. ▪ **Ever wonder what's in those TV dinners you heat up in the oven?** Hidden sugars galore, unfortunately (not to mention hydrogenated oils and questionable preservatives), even in the "healthy" brands. The only meat-containing frozen dinners I can recommend are Shelton's whole-wheat chicken or turkey potpies, both of which are sugar-free.

GO FISH

210. ▪ **Fried fish is a no-no** for many reasons, not the least of which is that the batter that coats the fish usually contains white flour and white sugar. Better to go for baked, broiled, or poached fish instead or . . .

211. ▪ **Make your own batter and oven-"fry" fish.** Dipping fish in an egg wash or oil and then coating it with whole-grain flour, ground-up nuts or seeds, and a variety of herbs makes for a much tastier breading, and you won't even miss the hidden sugar normally found in this entrée. This recipe comes from *Super Immunity for Kids* by Leo Galland, M.D.:

▪ OVEN-"FRIED" FISH ▪

$\frac{1}{2}$ cup milk *or* 1 beaten egg
$\frac{1}{4}$ teaspoon tarragon
$\frac{1}{2}$ cup whole-wheat bread crumbs *or* cornmeal
$\frac{1}{2}$ teaspoon paprika
$\frac{1}{2}$ teaspoon Parmesan cheese
$\frac{1}{4}$ teaspoon dry mustard
$2\frac{1}{2}$ pounds fish fillets
Lemon juice to taste
Sprigs of parsley for garnish

Preheat oven to 475 degrees. Lightly oil a cookie sheet or baking dish large enough to hold the fillets side by side. In a bowl large enough to fit the fillets, combine the milk or beaten egg and tarragon. In another bowl, mix the bread crumbs or cornmeal, paprika, Parmesan cheese, and mustard. Dip each fillet into the liquid mixture, then roll it in the seasoned bread crumbs or cornmeal. Place the fillets on the cookie sheet or baking dish. Bake for 7 to 10 minutes, until the fillets turn golden brown and are just done. Squeeze fresh lemon juice on top and garnish with parsley. *Serves 4 to 5 people.* ▪

Note: The time needed to cook fish will vary depending on the thickness of the fish. As a general rule, ten minutes of baking is needed per inch of fish thickness.

212. ▪ **A wedge of lemon and a few herbs such as dill and parsley** are often the very best condiments for topping fish. It's an added bonus that they just happen to be low in sugars.

213. ▪ **Eating cold-water fish rich in omega-3 essential fatty acids (EFAs)** is good for health in general, but it may be particularly helpful for diabetics. Omega-3 EFAs supplied by fish are believed to increase the efficiency of insulin because some studies show that diabetics who take omega-3 EFAs are able to decrease their dosage of insulin. Although more studies need to be done, I recommend that most of my clients eat cold-water fish rich in omega-3 EFAs at least once a week. Omega 3-rich fish include salmon, tuna, trout, mackerel, sardines, cod, and herring.

214. ▪ **Convenient frozen-fish products** to have on hand when you don't want to cook are Salmon Medallions, Halibut Medallions, and Tuna-Pesto Medallions from Northwest Naturals. (They're all sugar-free.)

215. ▪ **And what could be more convenient than canned tuna?** Open up a can for a meal anytime, anywhere, for a great source of blood-sugar-stabilizing protein.

216. ▪ **Don't forget about shellfish** such as shrimp and scallops. They are powerhouses of minerals, such as zinc, that are balancing to the blood sugar.

POINTS TO PONDER ABOUT PASTA

217. ▪ **If you've been piling the pasta on your plate** in an effort to get the fat out of your diet and off your body, you may unknowingly be sabotaging your effort. So says a February 8, 1995, article in the *New York Times:* "So It May Be True after All: Eating Pasta Makes You Fat." High-carbohydrate meals such as those centered around refined pasta cause the pancreas to secrete insulin, a fat-storage hormone par excellence. For the increasing number of people who are becoming insulin resistant, eating too many carbohydrates such as pasta can be disastrous— not only helping to keep the weight on but also increasing susceptibility to such diseases as diabetes and heart disease.

218. ▪ **Don't forget that the commercial pasta** you buy in supermarkets and get in restaurants is made from wheat that has had most of its nutrients stripped away. Although it has some B vitamins and iron added back in, white pasta is missing all the other nutrients important for proper blood-sugar function—especially chromium, manganese, and zinc.

219. ▪ **Try not to make pasta the cornerstone of your meal.** Use it as a side dish instead, and replace white pasta with the whole-wheat variety. Whole-wheat spaghetti still raises the blood sugar more than whole grains do (because it's more processed than whole grains), but its higher nutrient and fiber content make it a much better choice for your blood sugar and your health than white pasta.

220. ▪ **If you don't like whole-wheat spaghetti,** try brown-rice spaghetti, a mild, versatile, whole-grain pasta that's better liked than whole-wheat spaghetti by people who are used to refined pasta.

221. ▪ **Or try pasta made from spelt,** an unusual-sounding grain that is regarded as a delicacy in Germany and other parts of Europe. With its pleasant, almost nutty flavor, spelt pasta is a well-loved, nutritious addition to the diets of people who have come to realize that white pasta is not in the best interests of their blood sugar. If you'd like to try spelt pasta, look for an assortment of pasta shapes and sizes by Vita-Spelt.

222. ▪ **As the name implies, spaghetti squash is a perfect substitute for spaghetti.** The next time you make an Italian pasta or pesto sauce, try using baked spaghetti squash in place of pasta. To make enough for four main-course entrées or six side dishes, follow my easy squash recipe:

▪ ▪ ▪

▪ BAKED SPAGHETTI SQUASH ▪

1 large spaghetti squash or 2 small spaghetti squash
Italian tomato sauce or pesto sauce

Deeply pierce the skin of the squash in several places with a fork and place in a baking dish. Preheat oven to 375 degrees and bake the squash for 25 minutes, or until the skin is soft to the touch. Let the squash cool for 10 minutes, then cut in half lengthwise. With a spoon, remove the seeds and strings from the center of the squash, then fluff up the flesh with 2 forks until you have spaghettilike strands. Transfer to serving plates and top with sauce. *Makes 4 main-course entrées or 6 side dishes.* ▪

223. ▪ **Or use steamed shredded zucchini in place of pasta.**

AMBER WAVES OF GRAINS AND BEANS

224. ▪ **When eaten in moderation, unrefined whole grains** can go a long way toward balancing your blood sugar. Don't forget that complex carbohydrates such as these release their sugars slowly and gradually in the system, the way that is best for your sugar-handling mechanisms. In addition, whole grains that have their bran and germ intact are chock-full of blood-sugar-regulating nutrients and fiber.

225. ▪ **Use brown rice instead of white rice.** Brown rice has such a delightful flavor and chewy texture that most people wonder why they ever ate white rice to begin with. To make it, add 2 cups of water or stock and 1 cup of brown rice in a saucepan, heat it to a boil, then turn the heat down and let it simmer for 40–50 minutes (usually 40 minutes for short-grain and 50 minutes for long-grain).

226. ▪ **If you live life in the fast lane,** use quick-cooking brown rice. It's a snap to make, and it's becoming available from several different companies. Two brands I like are Arrowhead Mills Instant Brown Rice and Lundberg Farms Quick Brown Rice.

227. ▪ **Try other whole grains for variety.** All are packed with nutrition, and each one has a special taste all its own. If you're not familiar with whole grains, here are a few you should get to know:

> *Brown Basmati Rice:* a brown-rice cousin that has a delightful popcornlike aroma and is particularly good in Indian dishes.
>
> *Barley:* a chewy whole grain used primarily in soups, but it's delicious as a side dish for beef and lamb dishes as well.
>
> *Millet:* a gluten-free grain that has a pleasant, slightly nutty flavor.
>
> *Quinoa:* pronounced "keen-wa." A strange-sounding food that's not in the grain family but is often called a super-grain because it's packed with nutrition and is a complete source of protein all on its own. Its light flavor goes well in soups, salads, and pilafs.

228. ▪ **Legumes such as beans and peas are not only low in fat,** they're low on the Glycemic Index as well. Although most legumes contain some naturally occurring sugars, they cause only a minimal rise in blood sugar. This is just one more reason you should eat them.

▪ BONUS TIP: *If you haven't eaten many beans before, try soaking dry beans overnight to make them more digestible, and start out eating small portions.*

229. ▪ **Blackstrap molasses is high in nutrients and sweetening power,** so a little bit in such dishes as sweet beans is all you need. The following recipe, from *Healing with Whole Foods* by Paul Pitchford, demonstrates this. *One Sweet Tooth.*

▪ BAKED SWEET BEANS ▪

2 cups soaked beans (adzuki, lima, navy, or kidney)
8–10 cups water
$\frac{1}{2}$ onion, chopped (optional)
1 tablespoon molasses
1 teaspoon dry mustard
$\frac{1}{4}$–$\frac{1}{2}$ teaspoon sea salt

Discard soaking water and place soaked legumes in a pot with fresh cold water. Place pot on top of the stove. Bring to a boil for 15 minutes to loosen skins. Pour legumes and water into a baking dish. Cover and place in a 350-degree oven for 3–4 hours. When beans are about 80 percent done, add the rest of the ingredients. Then return to oven and cook until soft. Remove the cover to brown. *Serves 6 to 8 people.* ▪

VEGETABLES SIDE AND CENTER

230. ▪ **"Have you had your vegetables today?"** That's a question you should ask yourself each and every day. High in antioxidants and fiber, vegetables are also low in sugars, fat, and calories. They're what nutritionists call "nutrient-dense foods." What more could you ask for? Eat them liberally, three to five times daily.

231. ▪ **Vegetables that are fresh and in season** taste great and don't cry out for seasoning of any kind, let alone some type of sweet sauce. Try growing your own or shopping in farmers' markets if you're so inclined, and buy organically grown produce when available. You're likely to taste the difference.

232. ▪ **Vary the veggies you eat** to keep your diet interesting. This is always important, but especially when your diet becomes more limited because you're avoiding sugar-rich foods. Actually, you should look at your new eating plan this way: When you get the sugar out of your diet, you're not so much giving up some kinds of foods as you are making room for more essential ones—such as vegetables.

233. ▪ **With or without meat,** stir-fried vegetables are a great (sugar-free) way to get even the staunchest vegetable avoiders to eat their veggies.

234. ▪ **Chinese five-spice powder, with its sweet, licoricelike taste,** is a delightful way to sweeten any stir-fry. Here's one delicious example from my book *Beyond Pritikin:*

▪ FIVE-SPICE CHICKEN AND VEGETABLE SAUTÉ ▪

½ cup chicken broth
2 whole chicken breasts (2 pounds chicken), skinned,
    boned, and cut into ½-inch pieces
2 stalks broccoli, lightly steamed and diagonally sliced
½ red bell pepper, sliced
2 carrots, lightly steamed and diagonally sliced
2 yellow crookneck squash, diagonally sliced (optional)
¼ cup sliced onion
¼ cup canned water chestnuts, drained and sliced
1 tablespoon chopped fresh parsley
¼ teaspoon Chinese five-spice powder
2 cups cooked brown rice

Heat chicken broth in a skillet or wok. Add chicken and cook until tender. Remove chicken from broth and set aside. Add broccoli, red bell pepper, carrots, squash, onion, and water chestnuts. Stir and cook 2 to 3 minutes. Add parsley, Chinese five-spice powder, and brown rice. Return cooked chicken to mixture. Stir until thoroughly heated. *Serves 4.* ▪

235. ▪ **If heating up a TV dinner is more your style** than cooking a vegetarian meal from scratch, you're in luck. Several companies now offer vegetarian frozen entrées such as lasagna, enchiladas, and macaroni and cheese that don't contain added sugar. Brands to look for include Amy's and Cedarlane, and Taj of India makes good vegetarian Indian entrées.

236. ▪ **A cooked sweet potato** is a great way to satisfy your sweet tooth. Full of fiber and nutrients, sweet potatoes also have another unexpected advantage: They rank only 48 on the Glycemic Index. That means you can enjoy their special sweet flavor without experiencing a drastic rise in your blood sugar.

237. ▪ **Here's some news that probably sounds too good to be true:** Eating your baked potato with a little butter, high-quality oil, sour cream, or low-fat cheese is better for your blood sugar than eating it plain. This tip might go against everything you've been led to believe, but here are the facts: A baked potato is a very high inducer of insulin. It ranks between 80 and 89 on the Glycemic Index. But eating fat or protein with that potato will slow down the insulin response and keep your blood sugar steadier.

238. ▪ **Eating sulfur-rich onions** may be normalizing to the blood sugar and especially good for diabetics. In studies in Israel, the sulfur-containing component in onion was found to lower blood sugar and raise the levels of insulin in the cells. For this reason, I recommend using onions often in such dishes as stir-fries, soups, and stews. Or try baking one for a delicious, simple side dish:

▪ BAKED SWEET ONION ▪

1 large Spanish onion per person (or Walla Walla, Vidalia, or Maui, if available)

Keep the skin on the onions intact. Place in a baking pan and bake at 400 degrees for 1 hour. To serve, remove the outer skins and slice off the root ends. *Serve 1 onion per person.* ▪

239. ▪ **Good things sometimes come in small, unexpected packages.** Such is the case with the little-used vegetable the Jerusalem artichoke. Also called sunchoke, this small, sweet, tuberlike vegetable contains naturally occurring FOS (see tip 71) and is a unique source of inulin, a hormonelike chemical that reduces insulin needs and may be particularly beneficial for diabetics. If you'd like to try Jerusalem artichokes, eat them raw by themselves, spread them with nut butter, or dip them in a dressing. You can also lightly stir-fry them with other vegetables or sauté them in a garlic-herb butter.

240. ▪ **Get to know the low-starch vegetables,** those that raise the blood sugar only slightly. If you are having trouble maintaining a balanced blood sugar or your proper weight, it may help to emphasize lean meats and the following low-starch vegetables: asparagus, green beans or wax beans, broccoli, brussel sprouts, cabbage, cauliflower, celery, cucumbers, endive, kale, romaine or leaf lettuce, mushrooms, mustard greens, peppers, radishes, and spinach.

▪ ▪ ▪

A SAUCE FOR ALL SEASONS

241. ▪ **Sugar- and salt-containing sauces** have a way of covering up the unpleasant taste of processed foods. It's my hunch that that's why sauces are used so much these days. Be sure to use a sauce on entrées for the right reason: to accentuate the flavor of the whole-food ingredients you're using, not to disguise the taste of lifeless refined foods.

242. ▪ **Make the sauce with unrefined foods, too.** Don't make the mistake of cooking fresh meat and fresh vegetables and then covering them up with a gravy made with all-purpose flour. Use a whole-grain flour instead.

▪ BONUS TIP: *Powdered arrowroot or kudzu root also work well as thickeners. Dissolve a tablespoon of one of them in liquid and add during the last five minutes of simmering your sauce.*

243. ▪ **Or use a tablespoon of peanut butter** for a whole new taste. Peanut butter adds more protein and minerals to a sauce than flour and also imparts extra richness and creaminess.

244. ▪ **Sometimes a little spice is nice.** That's when Indian sauces such as those from Geetha's Gourmet or Taj of India come in handy. With no refined sugar, and such varieties as Madras Herb and Bombay Almond, these simmer sauces can quickly transform any plain meat, beans, or vegetables of your choice into Indian cuisine.

245. ▪ **In Greek Tszitziki Sauce,** cucumber, herbs, and unsweetened yogurt combine to create a cooling contrast to the spicy beef, lamb, or chicken shish kebabs this sauce usually tops. With no sugar and such simple ingredients, the sauce is delightfully easy to make, too. (See tip 196 for the recipe.)

246. ▪ **Tabasco hot sauce** can splash a little south-of-the-border seasoning on your foods. Containing only cayenne, vine-

gar, and salt, Tabasco is a bold seasoning that is particularly
good on meats and Mexican dishes, and it's entirely sugar-free.

247. ▪ **The same holds true for salsa,** which is just as good
to dab on entrées and side dishes as it is to dip chips in.

248. ▪ **A dash of tamari soy sauce** is an easy, sugarless way
to give your foods a Chinese flair. Steer clear of teriyaki and
sweet-and-sour sauces, though; they're both made with sugar.

249. ▪ **Pasta sauce** can be an unexpected source of sugars.
This is surprising because the tomatoes from which pasta sauce
is made are naturally sweet. A brand such as Prego may adver-
tise that "it's in there," but I bet you didn't know that meant
corn syrup and *up to fifteen grams of sugars* were "in there." Look
for a brand that contains no added sugar (such as Millina's
Finest or Classico) or for one that has five grams of sugars or
less per serving (such as Organic Garden Valley).

250. ▪ **Or make your own without any added sugar.** Holly
Sollars, a natural-food recipe tester and developer from Tucson,
Arizona, reports that dry-sautéing flavorful vegetables produces
a naturally sweet sauce. Besides, pasta sauce always tastes better
when it's homemade, anyway. Here's Holly's recipe for Fresh
Pasta Sauce that utilizes this helpful tip. *One Sweet Tooth.*

▪ ▪ ▪

■ FRESH PASTA SAUCE ■

1½ teaspoons extra-virgin olive oil
1 medium red onion, diced
1 clove garlic, minced
¼ pound fresh mushrooms, sliced thin
2 tablespoons rosé wine (optional)
3–4 fresh medium tomatoes, peeled and diced or pureed*
1 15-ounce can of organic tomato sauce
1½ tablespoons minced fresh basil leaves (or 2 teaspoons
     dried basil leaves)
1½ teaspoons minced fresh oregano leaves (or ¾ teaspoon
     dried oregano leaves)
Pepper to taste

Put olive oil in pan, then sauté together the onion, garlic, and mushrooms, stirring constantly for one minute. Add the optional rosé wine, and sauté for a minute or two more. Then dice the peeled tomatoes or, for a sauce with a smoother consistency, puree tomatoes in a blender or food processor for no more than 10 seconds. Add the diced or pureed tomatoes to the sautéed mixture along with the tomato sauce, basil, oregano, and pepper. Simmer on low, covered, for 30–45 minutes. *Makes about 4 cups.* ■

251. ■ **Pesto sauce** is a great example of how sauces made with natural ingredients are truly delectable without sugar of any kind. Made with fresh basil, parsley, nuts, garlic, Parmesan cheese, olive oil, and lemon, pesto sauce is great on vegetables,

---

*To peel tomatoes, make an *X* at the blossom end of each tomato with a paring knife. Core the other end. Place the tomato in boiling water for 30–40 seconds. Remove from the boiling water and place in ice-cold water until cold to the touch. Pull skin off each tomato.

whole-grain pasta, and whole grains such as brown rice. When you don't have time to make this traditional fresh basil sauce at home, use a commercial brand such as Rising Sun Farms Pesto Sauce to help you make a quick dinner.

252. ▪ **This Green Herb Sauce** also tops grains and pasta well. It's good on fish, too. It was developed by Deborah Madison for Dr. Gene Spiller's book, *Eat Your Way to Better Health.*

▪ **GREEN HERB SAUCE** ▪

(Salsa Verde)
1 cup parsley leaves, finely chopped
2 small garlic cloves, minced
1–2 tablespoons capers, rinsed and chopped
1 shallot, finely diced
¾ cup extra-virgin olive oil
Salt to taste
Juice of 1 large lemon to taste

Combine everything but the lemon juice in a bowl. Just before using, add lemon juice to taste. *Makes 1½ cups.* ▪

253. ▪ **A few tablespoons of barbecue sauce** can make a sugar-free entrée of fish, meat, or fowl suddenly turn into the sugar equivalent of a heavily sweetened dessert. Whether they're sweetened with sugar, brown sugar, corn syrup, honey, molasses, or fruit juice, commercial barbecue sauces are just too sweet to recommend in their straight form. If you must buy a commercial sauce, check the labels and look for the lowest-sugar version you can find. Then lower its sugar content even more by diluting it with water before you serve yourself or marinate your food.

254. ▪ **Or make this ultraquick barbecue sauce** from *Allergy Cooking Tricks and Treasures* by Nancy Burrows. *One Sweet Tooth.*

▪ WHIZZED BARBECUE SAUCE ▪

1 medium tomato, peeled, *or* 6 to 8 cherry tomatoes
2 pineapple rings (unsweetened, canned) *or* about 8
    chunks
1 tablespoon fresh lemon juice
1 tablespoon green onion (optional)
1 teaspoon dry mustard (optional)

Process ingredients in the blender. It's ready to use on any meat, fish, or fowl. *Makes enough sauce for 4 large chicken breasts.* ▪

CHAPTER 5

Get the Sugar Out
of Sandwiches and Snacks

Sandwich fixings, condiments, and snacks offer the ultimate in convenience. Little fuss, little preparation time, and food at our fingertips.

The quick simplicity of these products sometimes sounds too good to be true—and it is. We're paying a price for these packaged products in the form of hidden sugars, which add up in calories (and, eventually, in excess weight).

At first glance, the sugar content of cold cuts, condiments, and easy-to-grab snack foods doesn't seem like that big a deal. But a gram of sugar here, a few grams of sugar there, and five grams of sugar there eventually add up. Before you know it, you consume as much sugar (and calories) in one serving of snack foods as you do eating a rich, sugary dessert. Little by little, day after day, these seemingly insignificant sugar sources increase in number and take their toll on our overworked sugar-balancing systems.

Getting the sugar out of sandwiches and snacks does not mean the end of convenience. Some easy-to-use commercial products fit nicely into a low-sugar way of life, and this chapter will point them out. Also, some recipes (such as the one for Pizza Muffins in tip 272) can be ultimate time-savers. If you make a batch of these and freeze them, you have truly fast food that's both nutritious and low in sugars.

Last, remember that you get a great bonus when you get the sugar out of sandwiches and snacks and use fresh ingredients instead. The taste of these foods measurably improves and becomes much more satisfying.

SANDWICH FIXINGS

255. ▪ **High-quality whole-grain bread** can make your sandwich special. Review the "Breads and Spreads" section in chapter 2 if you need a refresher course on how to pick out this crucial sandwich component.

256. ▪ **Steer clear of cold cuts,** those convenient sandwich fillers that have the nasty habit of containing unwanted sugars and additives. Use instead:

257. ▪ **Leftover roast chicken, turkey, or roast beef slices,** which are, of course, sugar-free. Finish your sandwich off with red-onion slices, red-leaf lettuce, and a dab of gourmet mustard and you will have a sandwich fit for a king or queen.

258. ▪ **Or use flaked canned tuna or salmon.**

259. ▪ **Or hard-boiled egg slices** and a potpourri of healthy vegetables such as avocado and tomato slices, green pepper strips, and spinach leaves.

260. ▪ **Definitely spread your bread with unsweetened peanut butter** (or any other unsweetened nut butter), but skip the jelly. For a real treat, try thin apple or pear slices on your sandwich in place of jelly. *One Sweet Tooth.*

261. ▪ **Or nut butter with shredded or scraped carrot for a sandwich filling.** *One Sweet Tooth.*

262. ▪ **Bean spreads** are relatively new offerings on the market but nice vegetarian alternatives to the usual sandwich fare. Watch out for sweetened, fat-free bean spreads, however. Like many other fat-free foods, these products now have sugar in place of fat.

CONDIMENTS TO RELISH

263. ▪ **Choose your condiments with care** and go over those labels with a fine-tooth comb. Small amounts of sugars tend to creep into everything from mayo to relish and gradually add up. Remember, if you have a tablespoon of mayo and a tablespoon of ketchup on your burger, you consume *six grams of unnecessary sugars.* I personally prefer to skip these condiments altogether and occasionally treat myself to a cookie with six grams of sugars instead.

264. ▪ **Hold the salt** for a couple of reasons. First, too much salt in the diet can cause sugar cravings (as explained in tip 36). Second, commercial salt contains dextrose, which is another crafty way of saying table sugar.

265. ▪ **Understand that salt and sugar tend to go hand in hand in condiments.** The more manufacturers add of one, the more they add of the other—and our taste buds lose track of how much of both of them we taste. This is why many condiments, such as ketchup and barbecue sauce, contain more sugar than some desserts but we don't perceive them as being that sweet.

266. ▪ **Pass up the commercial ketchup,** a little something that seems so innocent but is really a sugar monger in disguise. In every tablespoon of ketchup, you get *a whole* *teaspoon of sugar.* In fact, ounce for ounce, ketchup has more sugar in it than ice cream!

267. ▪ **If your meal won't be complete without your favorite red spread,** seek out Westbrae Natural Unsweetened Un-Ketchup. Feel free to use a tablespoon of this ketchup on burgers and such without guilt. It's sugar-free. *One Sweet Tooth.*

268. ▪ **Become a mustard connoisseur.** Whether you use regular, stone-ground, Dijon-style, or horseradish-spiked, mustard is one condiment that is almost always sugarless. Have fun experimenting with different varieties of this pungent spread in a variety of ways. (It goes without saying, however, that you should continue to read the labels of the mustards you buy. You never know when manufacturers might decide to add sugar.)

269. ▪ **When a tablespoon of mayonnaise is what your sandwich needs,** make sure to use a brand, such as Spectrum Naturals, that contains no refined sugar. Try either Spectrum's Canola Mayonnaise, which is sweetened with honey and contains only one gram of sugar per tablespoon, or its Low-Cholesterol Mayo Spread, which is sugar-free. *One Sweet Tooth.*

270. ▪ **Or make your sandwich Italian-style:** Dress it with oregano and a vinegar-and-oil dressing for a new approach to your usual lunch.

THE SNACK CART

271. ▪ **Avoid eating sweets between meals.** Sure, we all get the munchies, but satisfying this need with sugary snacks is extremely stressful to the body (not to mention hard on the teeth). A satisfying snack will tide you over and keep you alert and energetic until your next meal. In-between-meal sweets don't meet that definition. Try instead more substantial mini-meals such as:

272. ▪ **A meal-in-a-muffin,** like one of the Pizza Muffins in this recipe or one of the Zesty Black Bean and Rice Mini-Muffins in tip 304. A meal-in-a-muffin is both a novel idea and term coined by cookbook author Jane Kinderlehrer in her book *Smart Muffins.* It is one of the most innovative coping strategies I know of to help you get the sugar out of your diet. If you have a supply of these in your freezer, you have complete, ready-to-eat, sugar-free meals at your fingertips—good for snacking or for breakfasts or lunch on the run. This handy recipe is one of many in *Smart Muffins.*

▪ PIZZA MUFFINS ▪

1 egg
½ cup tomato sauce
1 cup buttermilk or yogurt
4 slices mozzarella cheese, diced
¼ teaspoon freshly ground pepper
1 teaspoon crushed dry oregano
¼ teaspoon garlic powder
1½ cups whole-wheat pastry flour
3 tablespoons wheat germ
2 teaspoons baking powder
1 teaspoon baking soda
sliced tomato and cheese for garnish
sesame seeds

In a mixing bowl or food processor, blend together the egg, tomato sauce, and buttermilk or yogurt. Add the cheese and the spices. In another bowl, mix together the pastry flour, wheat germ, baking powder, and baking soda. Preheat the oven to 400 degrees. Butter or oil 12 regular-size muffin cups. Combine the two mixtures and mix until no flour is visible. Spoon the batter into the muffin cups and top each muffin with a slice of tomato, cover it with cheese, and sprinkle sesame seeds on top. Bake for 20–25 minutes. *Makes 12 muffins.* ▪

Or try:

273. ▪ **Low-fat cheese on whole-grain crackers** such as whole-wheat matzo or such Scandinavian flatbreads as Kavli or Ryvita.

274. ▪ **Vegetable "chips" and dip.** Cut up vegetables such as carrots, celery, jicama, and green pepper into stick or chip shapes and serve with a low-sugar dip such as the Greek Tszitziki Sauce in tip 196 or the Cottage Cheese Ranch Dip in tip 294.

275. ▪ **Celery spread with nut butter**—a quick, crunchy treat.

276. ▪ **Unsweetened bean spreads on whole-grain tortillas or chapatis.**

277. ▪ **Half a turkey or tuna sandwich,** on whole-grain bread, of course.

278. ▪ **An improvised mini-meal made from leftovers.** Here's one example: Reheat leftover brown rice, coat it with sesame or sunflower butter, and top with a few pieces of chopped dried fruit and a dash of cinnamon. *One Sweet Tooth.*

279. ▪ **Nuts, a natural for nibbling,** but be careful which types you consume. The honey-roasted varieties obviously are high in sugar, but did you know that sugar is often used in dry-roasting as well? If you've been eating dry-roasted nuts to lessen your fat intake, you've probably been eating hidden sugar instead. Here's a way to avoid extra fat and sugar: Home-toast raw nuts. Simply spread shelled raw nuts of your choice on a cookie sheet and bake at 275 degrees for 5–15 minutes (depending on the size of the nuts). The nuts are both nutritious and delicious.

280. ▪ **Low-sugar granola or granola bars.** Be especially careful with this suggestion. Most granola products on the market are cookies disguised as health food. The homemade granola in tip 150 and the granola bar below, however, are delicious exceptions that can work nicely as snacks (or for on-the-go breakfasts). *One Sweet Tooth.*

▪ ALMOND-OAT SQUARES* ▪

2 cups rolled oats
$1/2$ cup chopped or sliced almonds
$1/4$ cup oat bran
$1/4$ cup sesame seeds
Pinch of salt (optional)
$2/3$ cup applesauce or mashed banana
$2/3$ cup almond butter, room temperature

Combine the dry ingredients in a large bowl. In a small bowl, mix together the applesauce or mashed banana and the almond butter until well blended. Scrape the almond butter mixture into the oat mixture, mix well, then pat into an 11-by-7-inch baking dish. Bake at 300 degrees for about 35 minutes. Score with a knife while warm, then cut into square or bar shapes when cool. *Serves four.* ▪

Note: For a variation, use chopped peanuts and peanut butter or chopped cashews and cashew butter in place of the almonds and almond butter.

281. ▪ **If the above recipe isn't sweet enough for you,** here's one that should do the trick. Pumpkin puree in this recipe

*This recipe was adapted from a recipe for Sesame-Oat Squares in *The Yeast Connection Cookbook* by William G. Crook, M.D., and Marjorie Hurt Jones, R.N.

packs a nutritional punch and helps produce an especially tasty granola bar. This is another one from Jane Kinderlehrer, from her book *Smart Breakfast. Two Sweet Teeth.*

▪ PUMPKIN GRANOLA BARS ▪

¾ cup pumpkin puree
1 egg
¼ cup butter, at room temperature
¼ cup honey
2 tablespoons molasses
2 cups rolled oats
½ cup chopped peanuts, walnuts, or sunflower seeds
2 tablespoons shredded, unsweetened coconut
¼ cup wheat germ
½ teaspoon ground cinnamon
1 tablespoon grated orange rind

In mixing bowl or food processor, blend together the pumpkin, egg, butter, honey, and molasses. Add the oats, nuts, coconut, wheat germ, cinnamon, and orange rind, and process until ingredients are well combined. Spread mixture into a lightly greased 15½-by-10½-inch jelly-roll pan. Bake in a 350-degree oven for 40 minutes or until golden brown. While still warm, cut into 3-by-1½-inch bars. For very crisp bars, remove from pan to wire rack and cool completely. *Makes 30 bars.* ▪

CHAPTER 6

Get the Sugar Out
of Drinks and Party Foods

Most people seem to forget that beverages are part of their diets, too. Even when they watch their diets carefully, many Americans will think nothing of having a large glass of juice with breakfast, a can of cola with lunch and for a snack, and an alcoholic drink with dinner. They fail to realize that these liquids alone can easily add up to *125 grams of sugars*—well over the amount that is known to significantly impair the immune system. They also forget that these drinks will add *an extra 500 calories a day* to their tally, very likely adding an extra pound to their body fat each week.

Drinks certainly don't have to add weight, though. They can be refreshing, thirst-quenching, and even slightly sweet without being significant sources of sugars and calories. The tips in this chapter will point you toward ways to get the sugar out of the drinks you consume, but the first thing to remember is that good old, sugar-free water is the best thirst quencher of all. Our bodies are more than two-thirds water, and every fluid and tissue that we have, from our blood to our bones, requires water to function properly. It's vital to understand that water is the only drink that's a nutrient all by itself—and something we should all drink more of. If you can make only one change in your diet, switching from drinking sugary soda to purified water will get significant sugar out of your diet and is one of the most health-promoting changes I can recommend.

Unlike beverages that we consume every day, party foods are reserved for special occasions. From what I've seen in my clients' food diaries, these special occasions often turn into sugary occasions. Hidden in some of the most basic party hors d'oeuvres and entrées are sugars galore, and the sugar grams escalate to hazardous levels when typical party and holiday desserts are served.

You don't have to be a party pooper or holiday scrooge by serving less sweet food. To have your guests raving, use the freshest ingredients possible combined with irresistible herbs in the hors d'oeuvres and entrées you serve. Your guests' taste buds will be so tantalized that no one will miss the sugar. Then, if you want to have a sweet end to your event, by all means serve a dessert—just make sure it's a healthy one.

As I see it, drinks and party foods are extras in life. If we neglect to choose the ones we consume with care, they can be significant sources of extra calories that put on extra weight. But if we know how to get the sugar out of them, drinks and party foods can be additional sources of health-promoting nutrients as well as special treats.

DRINKING TO HEALTH

282. ▪ **If you do nothing else to get the sugar out of your diet,** just get the sugar out of the beverages you consume. Drinks are such common sources of empty calories that they are usually the first area I look at when I'm counseling my clients.

283. ▪ **Begin by steering clear of soft drinks,** the greatest single contributor of sugar in our diets. (This is an obvious tip that you should know by now!) Soft drinks are harmful to your health in every way, shape, and form, whether you're talking about the *39 grams of sugars* in one can of Coke, the phosphoric acid that throws your calcium balance out of whack, or the caffeine that continually stresses your adrenal glands. As the authors of *Eating for A's* said in their book, the sugar content of soft drinks makes them nothing more than "liquid candy bars with fizz."

284. ▪ **Diet drinks are dangerous** and definite no-no's even when you're trying to avoid sugar. (See tips 48–58 for more explanation.) Not only are aspartame-sweetened drinks believed to deplete the body of chromium, a mineral important for proper blood-sugar functioning, but the aspartame in these drinks may also break down on hot summer days into toxic chemicals that can cause a multitude of health problems. Some evidence now exists that the Desert Storm syndrome, an unexplained illness that affected thousands of Desert Storm soldiers, may have been caused by this phenomenon.

285. ▪ **The easiest substitute for soda** is juice mixed with sparkling mineral water. This drink still contains natural sugars, but it has less sugar than soft drinks and certainly more vitamins and minerals. Watch out for premade juice-and-sparkling-water combinations, though. Many of these drinks appear healthful but actually have such ingredients as sugar and high-fructose corn syrup, which turn the drinks into high-priced sodas. Far better for you to make this drink yourself so you can control the amount of sugar you ingest. Usually *Two Sweet Teeth.*

286. ▪ **Homemade ginger ale** is not only more tasty, more nutritious, and far lower in sugar than most ginger ales, but it's also a snap to make with the help of a wholesome product called Ginger Wonder Syrup by New Moon Extracts. Developed by master herbalist Paul Schulick, Ginger Wonder Syrup contains only pure Vermont honey and juiced, dried, and macerated organic ginger. A highly regarded tonic herb, ginger has natural anti-inflammatory properties, is good for digestive upset, and may in fact have blood-sugar-balancing properties. To make this healthful alternative to soda, just mix one teaspoon or less of Ginger Wonder Syrup in eight ounces of sparkling mineral water. What could be simpler? Look for this product in your local health-food store or call 1-800-543-7279 to find a store in your area that carries it. *Two Sweet Teeth*.

287. ▪ **Use stevia to make great-tasting sweet drinks.** The rest of the world has already caught on to this tip. In Japan, for example, artificial sweeteners such as aspartame and saccharin have been banned due to their probable adverse effects on health, but the Japanese aren't missing out on dietetic sodas. Drinks made with stevia are used by the thousands, and no adverse side effects have been reported. (See tip 70.) *Body Ecology Diet* author Donna Gates tells me that the following beverages made with stevia satisfy *Candida albicans* sufferers' desire for something sweet without aggravating their symptoms. Here's her most refreshing and welcome recipe. *One Sweet Tooth*.

▪ DONNA GATES'S LEMONADE OR CRANBERRY COOLER ▪

½ cup fresh lemon juice *or* ⅓ cup cranberry juice
  concentrate
⅛ teaspoon white stevia powder
4 cups cold water or chilled carbonated water

Mix the juice and stevia together until the stevia is completely dissolved. Add the water and serve the drink. *Makes about 4 servings.* ▪

288. ▪ **Make an iced herbal tea.** With so many varieties ranging from fruit-flavored to mint blends, herbal tea can delight just about anyone's taste buds. If you don't like tea plain, try adding just a pinch of the herb stevia or a drop of white stevia-powder liquid concentrate to sweeten the tea. *One Sweet Tooth.*

289. ▪ **Another refreshing treat** is to serve sparkling mineral water over ice cubes made from unsweetened natural fruit juices. With this tip you can make colorful drinks that have a touch of fruit sweetness without an excess of sugar. *One Sweet Tooth.*

290. ▪ **Avoid alcohol, which acts like pure sugar in the body** as well as a drug that taxes the liver and causes great nutrient deficiencies and imbalances. Many alcoholics are hypoglycemic, and some doctors now believe that sugar imbalances are a causal factor in alcoholism. It may seem unsocial not to drink alcohol or to drink only occasionally, but it is increasingly accepted and it's one of the simplest things you can do to get the sugar out and maintain good health.

291. ▪ **If you do drink alcohol,** make sure to stretch your drink by diluting it with club soda, seltzer, or water and lots of ice. Alcohol acts like sugar and provides empty calories, so moderation is the key here.

292. ▪ **Tonic water may seem like a harmless drink,** but don't be fooled. For every 12 ounces of tonic water, you get a whopping *18 teaspoons of sugar!* Skip the tonic and start employing the next tip instead.

293. ▪ **Sparkling mineral water with a twist of lemon or lime** is your best choice for a sugar-free drink at a cocktail party. Seltzer or club soda also are sugar-free, but many brands are high in sodium. All of these drinks look so much like a regular alcoholic drink, most people won't know you're not drinking.

TAKE A DIP

294. ▪ **Somehow a party just doesn't seem complete without a good dip** served on a party tray with colorful veggies. Here's a dip that can substitute nicely for the usual ranch dip full of hidden sugars.

▪ COTTAGE CHEESE RANCH DIP* ▪

1 cup low-fat cottage cheese
1–2 tablespoons buttermilk
1 tablespoon fresh lemon juice
1 tablespoon minced chives or green onion tops
2 teaspoons parsley flakes
1/2 teaspoon each onion powder and garlic powder

Blend all the ingredients in a blender until smooth. Chill at least an hour before serving. *Makes 1¼ cups.* ▪

295. ▪ **For an even quicker dip,** use a sugar-free mixing packet such as those from The Spice Hunter. With easy-to-add ingredients and savory herbal combinations, these mixes can make dreamy dips for those who don't have any time to spare.

296. ▪ **Salsa, which rarely contains sugar, is a party favorite.** Serve it with strips of cheese-crisp corn tortillas for extrafun occasions.

297. ▪ **Don't forget about guacamole,** another Mexican medley of vegetable flavors. If you don't make it from scratch, be sure to buy a brand that doesn't have any added sugars.

*This recipe was adapted from the Cottage Cheese Caper recipe in *Deliciously Low* by Harriet Roth.

298. ▪ **Middle Eastern eggplant dip or chickpea-based hummus** are two other sugar-free crowd-pleasers. Serve them with whole-grain pita bread or chapatis.

APPETIZERS AND HORS D'OEUVRES

299. ▪ **Serve low-fat cheese chunks and hearty whole-grain crackers** such as Ryvita Sesame-Rye any time, even for spur-of-the-moment social occasions.

300. ▪ **Who can resist the smell of fresh-made garlic bread?** Just about no one that I know of. To make a healthier (but still irresistible) version of this appetizer that's usually made with refined French bread, follow these directions: Mince a few garlic cloves and herbs such as parsley, rosemary, or thyme. Mix the seasonings in four tablespoons of soft butter or a butter–olive oil combination. Spread on top of 10 thick spelt bread or multigrain bread slices and bake at 350 degrees for 10–15 minutes. (Or you can place them under the broiler for a few minutes.) The only word to describe this is *yum!*

301. ▪ **Barbecued chicken drumsticks or wingdings** don't have to be sugar-laden to be gobbled up by your guests. Just use the Whizzed Barbecue Sauce from tip 254 on them and dress up the sauce with hot cayenne or savory rosemary. *One Sweet Tooth.*

302. ▪ **Serve barbecued vegetable kabobs** with the same sauce. *One Sweet Tooth.*

303. ▪ **Or marinate vegetables** in a vinaigrette, arrange on kabob skewers, and broil. A few good veggies to include are pepper and onion chunks, sliced zucchini, whole mushrooms, and cherry tomatoes.

304. ▪ **Now here's a marvelous idea for a cocktail party:** Zesty Black Bean and Rice Mini-Muffins. This is another recipe from *Smart Muffins* by Jane Kinderlehrer.

▪ ZESTY BLACK BEAN AND
RICE MINI-MUFFINS ▪

1 cup cooked black turtle beans
1 cup brown rice
¼ cup chopped fresh parsley
½ teaspoon curry powder
1 clove garlic, crushed
1 tablespoon tamari soy sauce
1 small egg
2 tablespoons sunflower seeds ground to a flour
½–¾ cup sesame seeds

In a mixing bowl, combine all the ingredients except the sesame seeds. Mix well with a fork. Preheat oven to 350 degrees and line a 2-dozen mini-muffin tin with paper liners. Form the mixture into walnut-size balls and roll in the sesame seeds. Place the balls in the muffin cups and bake for 10–15 minutes. These can be served hot or cold. *Makes two dozen mini-muffins.* ▪

305. ▪ **Meatballs are versatile hors d'oeuvres** for all occasions. Why are they so versatile? You can make them with either ground turkey, chicken, lamb, or beef—and you can top them with all kinds of low-sugar sauces ranging from Swedish-style sauce to pesto sauce to the Pasta Sauce in tip 250. Finally, they're popular with all kinds of people. What more could a host ask for?

306. ▪ **Talk about versatile!** Mini–shish kebabs certainly fit that description. They can be made with chicken, turkey, lamb, beef, shrimp, scallops, or even a firm fish such as swordfish. To make them, marinate the pieces in a low-sugar salad dressing such as vinaigrette or lemon juice, olive oil, garlic, and oregano. Skewer them on wooden sticks that have been soaked in water for at least 30 minutes, then broil.

■ BONUS TIP: *For the best flavor, marinate meats overnight in the refrigerator. There's no need to do this with seafood and fish, though. They're so delicate that they don't do well with this extra tenderizing.*

307. ■ **For an Oriental flair,** make the same shish kebabs but marinate them in tamari soy sauce combined with sesame oil, fresh ginger, and garlic.

SPECIAL OCCASIONS

308. ■ **A party punch is one of the quickest ways I know of** to consume more sugar than my body can comfortably handle. With ingredients such as sugar, honey, ginger ale, and fruit-juice concentrates, most punches are sugar disasters waiting to happen. This one from *Sweet and Natural* by Janet Warrington isn't, because she cleverly thins out the sugar content of the juices with tea and adds aromatic sweet spices. Good served hot during the holidays or iced during the summer, a one-cup serving of this punch counts as one fruit exchange on the diabetic food exchange system. *One Sweet Tooth.*

■ ■ ■

▪ SPICED TEA ▪

2½ cups water
3 decaf tea bags (or 3 raspberry-leaf tea bags)
¼ teaspoon ground nutmeg
¼ teaspoon ground cinnamon
2 cups unsweetened apple juice
½ cup unsweetened orange juice
5 orange or lemon slices (optional)

Bring the water to a boil and steep the tea bags and the spices for 3 minutes. Remove the tea bags and stir in the apple juice and orange juice. If serving cold, pour the tea over ice and serve with an orange slice or lemon wedge. If serving hot, bring heat up until the tea simmers, add the orange or lemon wedges, and ladle the tea into mugs. *Serves 5.* ▪

309. ▪ **Festive fruit kabobs can be served as either a party appetizer or a fun dessert.** Arrange a variety of fresh fruit such as pineapple chunks, whole strawberries, banana slices, and melon balls on wooden skewers and see what a difference innovative food presentation can make. *One Sweet Tooth.*

310. ▪ **Or serve colorful fruit salad in a watermelon or pineapple boat.** This makes an unusually attractive sweet finish to any celebration. *One Sweet Tooth.*

311. ▪ **When a special occasion calls for an extraspecial treat,** make sure you use special, high-quality ingredients in place of refined sugar. Here's a good example from *The All-Natural Sugar-Free Dessert Cookbook* by Linda Romanelli Leahy. *Two Sweet Teeth.*

▪ ▪ ▪

▪ CHOCOLATE-COATED FRUIT PARTY PLATTER ▪

4 ounces unsweetened chocolate squares
1 tablespoon unsalted butter
½ cup unsweetened apple-juice concentrate
1 teaspoon natural vanilla extract
4 cups fresh fruit (whole strawberries, bananas, navel
    orange slices, kiwis, etc.)

Spray baking sheet with a vegetable cooking spray; set aside. In the top of a double boiler, over simmering water, melt chocolate and butter, stirring occasionally; remove from heat and cool slightly. Whisk in juice concentrate a little at a time until chocolate is smooth; add vanilla extract. If mixture is too thick, add a little more concentrate until it thins out. Dip ends of fruit into chocolate mix, twirling to coat lower half of each piece of fruit; let excess drip back into pan until all chocolate is used. Place fruit on prepared baking sheet; place in freezer 10 minutes to set chocolate. Refrigerate until ready to serve. *Makes 12 servings of 3 pieces each.* ▪

312. ▪ **A small serving of a rich dessert** is sometimes all you or your guests want. Here's a recipe for "real" cheesecake—miniature style. It's especially nice for entertaining. *Two Sweet Teeth.*

▪ ▪ ▪

▪ VERSATILE CHEESECAKE TARTS* ▪

Bottom Layer

⅓ cup sunflower seeds *or* almonds, ground fine
⅓ cup unsweetened coconut *or* whole-wheat honey
    graham-cracker crumbs

Filling

8 ounces of cream cheese
1 egg
2 tablespoons natural flavoring extract (use almond extract
    for amaretto cheesecake, lemon extract for lemon
    cheesecake, or vanilla extract for vanilla cheesecake)

Optional Topping

Sliced fresh fruit such as kiwi, strawberries, blueberries,
    raspberries, cherries, or peaches

Line the cups of two 12-muffin tins with paper liners. Combine the bottom layer ingredients and place one teaspoon of this mixture in the bottom of each liner. Press down with the back of a spoon to cover the bottoms. Preheat the oven to 325 degrees. To make the filling, cut the cream cheese into 8 blocks and blend with the other filling ingredients in a food processor, blender, or mixing bowl until smooth and creamy. Place a tablespoon of the filling in each tart cup and bake for 15 minutes. Top with fresh fruit slices if desired. *Makes 2 dozen tarts.* ▪

313. ▪ **"Have a happy, healthy birthday!"** That's what you'll be saying to the guest of honor when you present this

---

*This recipe was revised from a recipe for Amaretto Cheesecake Tarts in *Smart Cookies* by Jane Kinderlehrer.

wholesome cake instead of the usual store-bought variety. *Two Sweet Teeth.*

▪ EVERYTHING GOOD BIRTHDAY CAKE* ▪

1½ cups whole-wheat pastry flour
1 teaspoon baking powder
1 teaspoon baking soda
1 teaspoon ground nutmeg
pinch of salt
1 teaspoon ground cinnamon
⅓ cup melted butter or oil
½ cup fruit-juice concentrate
2 eggs, beaten
1 cup unsweetened applesauce

Preheat oven to 375 degrees. Combine dry ingredients. Combine liquid ingredients and add to dry. Mix well. (Note: Beating the egg yolks separately and adding to the wet ingredients, then folding in the beaten egg whites will produce a fluffier cake.) Pour mixture into a 9-inch cake pan and bake for 45 minutes, or until done. Allow to cool. Serve as is or add frosting of your choice from the "Icing on the Cake" section in chapter 7 if desired. *Serves 8 to 10 people.* ▪

314. ▪ **When sugar restriction is necessary for the birthday boy or girl,** just ask him or her to pick out the *absolute favorite allowable food* he or she can eat. Colorful candles can wish just as good tidings on strawberries and whipped cream, a muffin, or even on pizza as they can on a birthday cake, so don't

---

*This recipe was adapted from a recipe for Everything Good Birthday Cake that appeared in *Eating for A's* by Alexander Schauss, Barbara Friedlander Meyer, and Arnold Meyer.

get too tied to tradition. After all, a birthday party is designed to *celebrate the person*, not the food he or she can eat.

315. ▪ **Rethink your attitudes** surrounding birthdays, anniversaries, holidays, and other special occasions. Is it really necessary to have rich, gooey desserts to have a good time? The most festive, happy occasions usually involve just good entertainment and caring family and friends to share in the joyful experience. Don't lose sight of this.

HOLIDAY COPING STRATEGIES

316. ▪ *Moderation* **is the key word to keep in mind during the holidays.** Taste the special foods of the season, but don't go overboard. Especially try to avoid indulging in sugary foods during nonsocial occasions.

317. ▪ **Eat a protein-rich snack before you go to a party** where you know there will be lots of tempting desserts. A few pieces of chicken or turkey meat beforehand can keep you from being famished at the party and bingeing on too much sugar.

318. ▪ **If tired and stressed-out is how you usually feel** during the holiday season, avoid eating sweets and keep the meals that you make simple. Having ready-to-heat leftovers and sugar-free snacks on hand always helps.

319. ▪ **Continue to eat well-balanced meals and snacks** during the holidays. Doing so will balance your blood sugar and make you less likely to overindulge in holiday sweets.

320. ▪ **When you go on a long holiday shopping spree,** take high-protein snacks with you to sustain you. They'll keep you away from quick-fix sweets sold in shopping-mall food courts. Some good snacks to take are the Peanut Butter Muffins in tip 120, the Pizza Muffins in tip 272, or the Almond-Oat Squares in tip 280. Nuts are also good foods to carry along.

321. ▪ **Revise your typical holiday meal to lower its sugar content,** and be sure to substitute unrefined grain products for season-typical refined carbohydrates. Stuffing is okay—go ahead and enjoy a serving—just make sure it's made with whole grains or whole-grain bread instead of white bread.

322. ▪ **To replace sugar-rich canned cranberry sauce,** make this tangy, easy-to-fix, homemade version that's far superior in flavor. It was developed by Marjorie Hurt Jones, R.N., author of *The Allergy Self-Help Cookbook.* When it's cooking, the smell of the simmering cranberries, juice concentrate, and spices will drive your guests wild. *Two Sweet Teeth.*

▪ SPICY CRANAPPLE SAUCE ▪

1 pound fresh cranberries
1 to 1½ cups unsweetened apple-juice concentrate
½ teaspoon ground cinnamon
⅛ teaspoon ground cloves
1 tablespoon arrowroot
3 tablespoons water

Wash the cranberries carefully and discard any imperfect fruit. Place the berries, 1 cup juice concentrate, cinnamon, and cloves in a large saucepan. Bring to a boil, stirring occasionally. When bubbles first appear, reduce heat to low. Simmer for 10 minutes, or until most of the skins have popped. Taste the sauce. For a sweeter, juicier sauce, add the remaining ½ cup juice concentrate. Increase spices if desired. If sauce is too tangy, dilute with a little water. Dissolve the arrowroot in the 3 tablespoons of water. Stir into the hot berries. Cook, stirring, another 2–3 minutes, until thick and clear. Serve warm or cold. *Makes 1 quart.* ▪

323. ▪ **Candied sweet potatoes may be traditional,** but it's silly (and unhealthy) to add loads of concentrated, refined sweeteners to an already perfectly sweet food. Make this subtly sweet basic Sweet Potato Casserole instead for the holidays and everyone will leave satisfied. *One Sweet Tooth.*

▪ SWEET POTATO CASSEROLE ▪

6 large sweet potatoes
1 20-ounce can of unsweetened crushed pineapple, packed in juice
1 teaspoon ground cinnamon (optional)
1–3 tablespoons sesame oil (optional)
½ cup chopped pecans (optional)

Bake sweet potatoes on a cookie sheet at 375 degrees for about an hour, until done. Cut in half and scoop out the potato flesh. Discard the skin. Mash sweet potato with masher or with an electric mixer on low until smooth. Add pineapple, its juice, the cinnamon, and oil, and mix well. Spoon mixture into a lightly oiled casserole or a 9-by-13-inch baking dish. Sprinkle pecans on top if desired. Cover and bake for about 40 minutes. *Serves 10 to 12.* ▪

324. ▪ **If you have a traditional holiday recipe** that's been handed down through the ages, feel free to use it as long as you substitute Sucanat, date "sugar," or rice-syrup powder in place of the sugar the recipe may call for. (We know the facts about refined sugar better than they did in the good old days.)

325. ▪ **Pumpkin pie doesn't have to be terribly sweet to be pleasing.** This recipe will show you what I mean. *Two Sweet Teeth.*

▪ **PUMPKIN PIE*** ▪

1 teaspoon ground cinnamon
1/2 teaspoon ground ginger
1/2 teaspoon ground nutmeg
1/2 teaspoon ground cloves
1 1/2 cups pumpkin puree
1 cup milk
3 eggs, beaten
1/4 cup honey
1 1/2 tablespoons molasses
1 teaspoon natural vanilla extract

Preheat oven to 450 degrees. Add seasonings to pumpkin puree. In a large bowl, mix milk and eggs, then stir in pumpkin mixture, honey, molasses, and vanilla. Pour filling into the Whole Wheat Crust in tip 388 or into a store-bought, frozen whole-wheat crust such as the kind sold by Mother Nature's Goodies. Bake for 10 minutes, then reduce heat to 350 degrees and bake for 50 minutes longer. Cool on wire rack before serving. *Serves 8 to 10 people.* ▪

Note: In addition to the great taste of homemade pumpkin pie, the smell of pumpkin pie baking might just be an aphrodisiac for men. According to a study conducted by the Smell & Taste Treatment and Research Foundation in Chicago, the smells of pumpkin pie and lavender were the top arousing aromas for men.

*This recipe was adapted from a Pumpkin Pie recipe that appeared in *Rodale's Basic Natural Foods Cookbook* by Charles Gerras, editor, and the staff of Rodale Press.

326. ▪ Don't give refined, sugary sweets as gifts, and ask the same of others.

327. ▪ Keep the spirit of the season. Don't be so hung up on the foods and sweets of the season that you forget to enjoy what's most important: celebrating sweet, memorable times with those you love.

CHAPTER 7

Get the Sugar Out
of Baking, Desserts,
and Treats

My work with clients for more than twenty years has led me to conclude that most Americans fall into one of three types of dessert eaters—and none of these really know how to get the sugar out of their diets.

Type one is what I call the traditional dessert eater. This type indulges in desserts with a high fat and high refined-sugar content—foods such as cream pies, rich fudge, and butter cookies. The high fat content of these desserts is extremely satisfying and filling for traditional dessert eaters, but even the high fat content can't keep their excessive sugar consumption from taxing their blood-sugar-balancing mechanisms and causing them harm.

The second type is the natural-goodie dessert eater, also sometimes known as the health buff. This kind will eat anything as long as it's made with natural sweeteners and whole-grain flours. Health buffs are correct in part of their dessert philosophy—it is far better to consume goodies made with unrefined sweeteners and whole grains rather than those made with processed carbohydrates. Unfortunately, health buffs have conveniently forgotten about an equally important component of maintaining health—keeping the sugars one consumes, even the natural sugars, to an absolute minimum.

Type three, the fat-free-goodie eater, is the new kid on the block. Americans are converting to this type in droves because they have gotten some ill-conceived advice about fat. In a misguided attempt to avoid all fat, Americans who have embraced the fat-free philosophy are consuming more sugars than ever before, missing out on an essential nutrient (fat) that could help moderate their blood-sugar levels. As a result, increasing numbers of people are pigging out on fat-free foods they think are good for them and yet wondering why they are so tired, overweight, and disease-prone.

Although these three types of dessert eaters seem vastly different, they share one common bond—too much sugar in their diets. They all need to learn that moderation and balance among all nutrients is the key to healthy and enjoyable dessert eating. Most important, we all need to understand that the more we can cut down on sugars in the treats we consume, the better off our health will be.

Switching from enjoying a piece of cake with 25 grams of sugars to one with 5 grams is like going from A to Z. I wouldn't be honest or fair if I told you that you can make the switch overnight. You cannot. It has taken years for you to get used to the amount of sugars you currently consume in sweets, so be patient with yourself and realize that it's going to take a while to wean yourself away from all those sugars and to retrain your sweet tooth.

The tips in this chapter will show you practical ways to reduce the amount of sugars in the treats you buy and make. But overly sweetened desserts will forever tempt you until you develop a firm resolve about how vitally important it is to lower your sugar intake. If you start to forget just why you were getting the sugar out of your diet, copy the list of health problems associated with excessive sugar intake and put it up on your refrigerator. This should be an effective reminder of how much you need to consciously and persistently work at reducing your sugar intake each and every day—even in the desserts you consume.

Despite what you might believe, getting the sugar out of sweet treats does not mean eating tasteless desserts. I think you will be amazed at just how satisfying and special some of the minimally sweetened desserts in this section really are.

Even if some of the *One Sweet Tooth*–designated desserts initially seem too bland for your taste buds, you will be surprised at how much your taste buds can change. If you continue to eat less sugary foods, you will gradually but honestly come to prefer them, just as I have.

Treats are special simply because they are not something you have every day. But when you get the sugar out of the other areas of your diet, you may find that you can treat yourself a little more often to sweet indulgences as long as they are subtly sweetened, nutritionally balanced, and made with wholesome ingredients. The recipes and tips that follow emphasize the natural sweetness of fresh fruits and vegetables and *small amounts of natural sweeteners*. All of the following recipes avoid the denatured ingredients so common in popular American treats, and the goodness of the natural ingredients shines through in better taste and nutrition. It is my hope that these tips will stimulate your awareness and creativity to make desserts with life-giving foods full of nutrients.

We have all heard of desserts that are "to die for." This chapter will give you desserts to live for.

●●●

FABULOUS FRUITS

328. ▪ **Plain fresh fruit is a dessert all by itself.** What could be more delicious than a bowl of just-picked strawberries in the spring, a succulent piece of watermelon on a hot summer afternoon, or a crisp, juicy apple on an autumn day? Absolutely nothing as far as I'm concerned. "Just fruit" is just perfect for satisfying your sweet tooth naturally.

329. ▪ **Ripeness is the key** for enjoying fruit to its utmost. We've all tasted the difference between a mealy, bitter half of grapefruit and a juicy one that needs no sugar at all because it's perfect just the way it is. There's just no sense in buying fruit before (or after) its time.

330. ▪ **Get to know what's in season.** The availability and ripeness of fruits will vary from region to region, but the following chart gives some indication of when to buy produce at its prime. If you're ever in doubt, don't be afraid to ask the produce manager at your grocery store for his/her recommendations.

Apples: September–December
Apricots: June–August
Banana: Year-round
Blackberries: May–August
Blueberries: May–September
Cherries: June–August
Cranberries: October–December
Grapefruit: December–March
Grapes: August–November
Mangos: May–September
Melons: May–September

Oranges: December–March
Papayas: June–September
Peaches/Nectarines:
    June–August
Pears: November–February
Pineapple: March–June
Plums: May–October
Raspberries: May–July
Strawberries: April–July
Tangerines: November–February
Watermelon: May–August

▪ ▪ ▪

331. ▪ **Presentation is another key to enjoyment.** When you arrange fruit in a colorful and appetizing way, not only does the fruit taste better, but the whole experience becomes a whole lot "sweeter."

332. ▪ **Fresh fruit is tops in the taste department** and frozen fruit is second best. Canned fruit is a distant third. I recommend limiting the use of canned fruit, but if you buy it for convenience, be sure to buy it packed in its own juices or, better yet, in water. Canned fruit in heavy syrup has almost twice the sugar of the juice-packed variety.

333. ▪ **If you accidentally buy a syrup-sweetened can of fruit,** put the fruit in a strainer and rinse it well with filtered water. This will help send some of those extra sugars down the drain.

334. ▪ **Instead of putting sugar on top of half a grapefruit,** spread one teaspoon of olive oil over it. Then let it stand for several hours before serving. The oil will neutralize the acid in the grapefruit and increase its sweetness.

335. ▪ **For a new twist to an old staple,** serve honeydew melon with lime slices. Squeezing lime on it gives the melon a new, refreshing flavor.

336. ▪ **Rome Beauty, Golden Delicious, Jonathan, pippin, and Winesap** are all good baking apples. To make a baked apple (or a baked pear), preheat the oven to 350 degrees, core the fruit, fill it with the desired filling, and place 2 to 3 tablespoons of water in the baking dish with the fruit. Cover, or baste fruit with liquid several times during baking, and bake for 45–55 minutes, or until fruit is tender when pierced with a fork. Tasty, sugar-free filling ingredients to add include chopped walnuts or pecans; grated lemon or orange zest; cinnamon, nutmeg, cloves, or allspice; vanilla extract; or mint extract for a refreshing change of pace. *One Sweet Tooth.*

337. ▪ **For a slightly sweeter filling,** try adding one tablespoon unsweetened apple juice; or a teaspoon of maple syrup and half a teaspoon of maple extract; or one tablespoon of raisins, currants, or chopped dates; or one tablespoon of date "sugar"; or one tablespoon of plain, low-fat yogurt combined with one teaspoon of honey, a few drops of vanilla, and a dash of cinnamon. *Two Sweet Teeth.*

338. ▪ **When your taste buds want something new,** treat yourself to a fruit you haven't tried before. Some boysenberries, a guava, kiwi, or starfruit are exotic ways to break up your routine.

339. ▪ **Fruits vary in portion size because of their water and sugar contents.** Fruits with a lot of water (such as strawberries and watermelon) have a larger serving size (and also rank lower on the Glycemic Index) than fruits with less water such as bananas and dried fruits. As wonderful and vitamin-packed as fruit is, don't go overboard eating it. Remember that fruit is still a source of sugars even though it's a natural one. Limit yourself to no more than two to three of the following portions of fruit per day:

Apple—1 small
Apricots (fresh)—2 medium
Apricots (dried)—4 halves
Banana—1/2 small
Berries: boysenberries, blackberries,
    blueberries, raspberries—1/2 cup
Cantaloupe—1/4 (6-inch diameter)
Cherries—10 large
Dates—2
Figs (fresh)—1 large
Figs (dried)—1 small
Fruit cocktail (canned in juice)—1/2 cup
Grapefruit—1/2 small
Honeydew melon—1/8 (7-inch diameter)

Kiwi—1 medium
Mango—1/2 small
Nectarine—1 small
Orange—1 small
Papaya—3/4 cup
Peach—1 medium
Pear—1 small
Pineapple—1/2 cup
Plums—2 medium
Prunes—2 medium
Raisins—2 tablespoons
Strawberries—3/4 cup
Tangerine—1 large
Watermelon—1 cup

340. ▪ **An easy way to estimate the amount of fruit you're consuming** is to use your fist as a guide. The size of your fist equals about one cup of chopped fruit or one medium whole fruit.

FRUIT TOPPINGS

341. ▪ **Spreading unsweetened nut butter on apple, pear, or banana slices** is a way to enjoy these fruits but lessen their glycemic effects. This snack is a satisfying treat for anyone, but it is especially appreciated by diabetics and hypoglycemics. *One Sweet Tooth.*

342. ▪ **Toasted ground or slivered nuts or seeds** can also add a nice sugar-free finish to a bowl of fresh fruit. *One Sweet Tooth.*

343. ▪ **A few dashes of flavoring extract** can give fruit a dramatically new flavor, as you'll see in this easy recipe from *Beyond Pritikin. One Sweet Tooth.*

▪ VANILLA PEARS ▪

4 pears, cored, peeled, and halved (or fresh peaches, plums, or nectarines can be used when in season)
1 tablespoon water
1 teaspoon allspice
12 drops natural vanilla extract

Preheat oven to 325 degrees. Place pears and water in baking dish. Sprinkle with allspice and drizzle each pear half with 3 drops of vanilla extract. Cover and bake about 20 minutes. *Serves 4.* ▪

344. ▪ **The healthiest topping I know of** is unsweetened, low-fat yogurt with a pinch of FOS added to slightly sweeten it. (See tip 71 for more information about FOS.) Try this the next time you want something slightly sweet on fresh fruit. This topping is beneficial for almost everyone, but especially for individuals afflicted with yeast or parasitic infections or any type of digestive upset. The yogurt supplies friendly bacteria for the digestive tract, and the FOS feed the beneficial bacteria and help them multiply and thrive. *One Sweet Tooth.*

345. ▪ **Other yogurt topping ideas** include mixing plain yogurt with ½ teaspoon vanilla extract and a dash or two of cinnamon, or with ¼ teaspoon almond extract and toasted chopped almonds, or with ¾ teaspoon coconut extract and a tablespoon of unsweetened coconut. *One Sweet Tooth.*

346. ▪ **Creamy frosting,** such as the frostings in either tip 377 or 378, makes a delicious "dip" for fresh strawberries. *Two Sweet Teeth.*

347. ▪ **Serve your fruit Hawaiian style.** Top it with a tablespoon of unsweetened coconut milk. *One Sweet Tooth.*

348. ▪ **Or do as the British royalty do.** Serve berries with fresh cream. *One Sweet Tooth.*

349. ▪ **For special occasions,** serve fruit with whipped cream made with a teaspoon or two of honey instead of confectioners' sugar. *Two Sweet Teeth.*

350. ▪ **Pureed fresh fruit,** either by itself or combined with yogurt, makes a colorful and dressy topping for a fruit salad. In this recipe, Harriet Roth, author of *Deliciously Low,* shows us how to make an elegant dessert for a dinner party of fifteen without any fuss. *Two Sweet Teeth.*

▪ ▪ ▪

▪ LAST-MINTUE FRUIT MÉLANGE ▪

1 pint fresh strawberries, washed, then hulled
1 tablespoon frozen, unsweetened apple-juice concentrate
¼ cup plain yogurt
1 teaspoon natural vanilla extract
1 20-ounce package frozen, unsweetened peach slices
   (or fresh)
1 20-ounce package frozen, unsweetened blueberries
   (or fresh)
1 20-ounce package frozen, unsweetened bing cherries
   (or fresh)
2 bananas, peeled and sliced (optional)
Fresh mint sprigs for garnish

To make strawberry-yogurt dressing, place strawberries, juice concentrate, yogurt, and vanilla in blender or food processor. Process until pureed. Place in covered container in refrigerator until serving time. About 30 minutes before serving time, place frozen peaches, blueberries, and cherries in an attractive glass serving bowl. When ready to serve, add dressing to fruit and mix gently. Sliced bananas may be added at this time if desired. Garnish with sprigs of fresh mint and serve in glass coupes or small Chinese lotus bowls. *Serves 15.* ▪

VEG OUT FOR DESSERT

351. ▪ **Sweet, starchy vegetables** are ideal ingredients for making desserts without concentrated sweeteners. Such vegetables as sweet potatoes, winter squash, pumpkin, carrots, parsnips, Jerusalem artichokes, and beets all provide subtle sweetness chock-full of nutrients and fiber and can be used to make everything from substantial sweet breads to whipped mousse desserts.

352. ▪ **Use mashed butternut squash** as a base for pudding. This tip comes from Marjorie Hurt Jones, R.N., editor of the *Mastering Food Allergies* newsletter. To make this creamy pudding, use an electric mixer or food processor to mix the mashed pulp of one medium butternut squash with a few tablespoons of oil, a dash of cinnamon, and 1 to 1^1/$_2$ cups pureed seedless grapes, pineapple, or peeled pears. Pour the mixture into individual baking dishes, sprinkle chopped pecans on top if you wish, and bake at 350 degrees for about 20 minutes. *Serves 4. One Sweet Tooth.*

353. ▪ **Or serve baked winter squash with hot cinnamon syrup** for another delicious vegetable-based dessert. To make enough syrup for four servings, heat together 5 tablespoons of barley malt or rice syrup, 1 to 2 tablespoons butter, and a generous dash of cinnamon in a saucepan. Serve the squash with toasted nuts of your choice and pour the syrup on top. Remember, the butter and nuts in this dessert are good to include because their fat content helps slow down the body's response to the sweet syrup. *Two Sweet Teeth.*

354. ▪ **If you have a juicer gathering dust,** because you no longer use it, dust it off and start making vegetable juices again —to use in recipes. Experiment with using fresh carrot juice or carrot-beet juice in place of fruit-juice concentrates in recipes. This cuts the sugar and gives you a healthy dose of beta-carotene to boot.

355. ▪ **Here's an idea for a frozen parsnip dessert** that comes from my 106-year-old mentor, Dr. Hazel Parcells. *One Sweet Tooth.*

▪ ▪ ▪

▪ FROZEN PARSNIP DESSERT ▪

2 cups parsnips
1 pint heavy whipping cream
2 teaspoons honey
½ teaspoon natural vanilla extract
¼ teaspoon ground cardamom
Toasted walnut pieces (for garnish)

Thoroughly clean parsnips and freeze them in the freezer. While frozen, grate the parsnips or put them through a ricer so they will have the consistency of shredded coconut. Whip the whipping cream very stiff and add the honey, vanilla, and cardamom. Fold the grated parsnips into the whipped cream, pour into 4 individual serving glasses, top with toasted walnut pieces, and chill. *Serves 4.* ▪

TIPS FOR BETTER BAKING

356. ▪ **When a recipe calls for one cup of sugar,** use more nutritious Sucanat in equal amounts or, better yet, reduce the amount of Sucanat by one-third to one-half of the sugar called for in the recipe and use other dry ingredients in sugar's place.

357. ▪ **You also can use date "sugar"** instead of sugar in the same way.

358. ▪ **For a less sweet version of one of your favorite recipes,** use brown-rice syrup powder in equal proportions to the amount of sugar indicated.

359. ▪ **Fructose is sweeter than sugar;** one-third to two-thirds cup of fructose will give the same sweetening power as one cup of sugar. Use fructose primarily in chilled and frozen desserts. It tastes sweeter in cold dishes than in hot.

360. ▪ **To use liquid sweeteners in a recipe that calls for sugar,** substitute one-half to three-quarter cup of honey, maple syrup, molasses, or fruit-juice concentrate for one cup of sugar and decrease the other liquids in the recipe by one-quarter cup for each three-quarter cup of sweetener.

▪ BONUS TIP: *If your honey ever crystallizes, simply set the jar in a bowl of hot water and the crystals will dissolve.*

361. ▪ **You can also use one and a half cups of barley malt or rice syrup** in place of one cup of sugar and reduce the liquids in a recipe by one to two tablespoons.

▪ BONUS TIP: *To help sticky sweeteners such as barley malt or honey slip out of measuring spoons or cups, lightly oil your utensils or spray them with a nonstick cooking spray before using.*

362. ▪ **To use stevia in recipes,** use one-half to one teaspoon in place of one cup of sugar and add one to two tablespoons extra liquid. (For more about stevia, see tip 70.) Nicolette Dumke, author of *Allergy Cooking with Ease,* suggests using stevia in recipes that contain strongly flavored ingredients such as carob or cranberries because stevia has a slight licoricelike taste. She also warns that stevia-sweetened baked goods do not brown much, even when they're done. For that reason, you should time your baking carefully and check for doneness by touch.

363. ▪ **To cut down the amount of honey, maple syrup, molasses, or juice concentrate** in a recipe, reduce the amount of sweetener by half and substitute unsweetened applesauce or mashed sweet potato for the other half.

364. ▪ **Slash the sugar even further** by using all unsweetened applesauce, pureed fruit, or pureed sweet potatoes.

365. ▪ **Reduce it further still** by mixing half unsweetened applesauce or pureed fruit with half water or herbal tea. Stevia tea works well in these kinds of cases where the least amount of sweetening is desired.

366. ▪ **Rice milk, soy milk, almond milk, or amasake** are four other ingredients that can lend their subtle, creamy sweetness to recipes when you want to eliminate more concentrated sweeteners.

367. ▪ **Know the sugar content of the sweeteners you're considering using.** The following list gives you the grams of sugars in one tablespoon of each sweetener, rounded to the nearest half gram. Since brands sometimes vary in sugar content, some sweeteners have a range of grams of sugars listed.

Honey—16–18 grams (17 grams on average)
Fructose—12–15 grams
Blackstrap molasses—11–15 grams
Maple syrup—13 grams
Liquid FruitSource—11 grams
Granular FruitSource—7.5 grams
Apple juice concentrate—7.5 grams
Other juice concentrates—5.5–8.5 grams
All-fruit spread—1–12 grams (9 grams average)
Unsweetened apple butter—4–8 grams
Barley malt—6 grams
Brown-rice syrup—5 grams
Rice-syrup powder—4 grams
Sucanat—3 grams
Chatfield's date "sugar"—3 grams
Amazake brand amasake—2 grams
Unsweetened apple juice—2 grams
Other juices—1.5–2 grams
Unsweetened applesauce—1.5 grams
Other fruit-flavored applesauces—1.5 grams
Rice milk, soy milk, and almond milk—0.5–1 grams

368. ▪ **Use rose water or orange blossom water** in place of vanilla or in place of one teaspoon of sweetener to delicately flavor cakes and cookies.

369. ▪ **Don't just replace white sugar in a recipe;** replace white flour as well. For every cup of white flour called for, use seven-eighths cup of whole-wheat flour or whole-wheat pastry flour.

370. ▪ **Experiment with other nutritious whole-grain flours,** which can add new flavor and texture to your baked goods. For variety, try one of the following substitutions in place of one cup of whole-wheat flour:

> 1 cup of multigrain flour
> $1\frac{1}{3}$ cups ground rolled oats
> $\frac{5}{8}$ cup brown-rice flour plus $\frac{1}{2}$ cup rye flour
> $\frac{1}{2}$ cup potato flour plus $\frac{1}{2}$ cup rye flour
> $1\frac{1}{4}$ cups rye flour
> $\frac{3}{4}$ cup brown-rice flour plus $\frac{1}{3}$ cup amaranth flour
> 1 cup kamut flour
> 1 cup spelt flour

371. ▪ **Try substituting chestnut flour** in cake and cookie recipes in place of part of whatever flour you're using. Chestnut flour is a wholesome way of adding extra lightness, creaminess, and sweetness to baked goods.

HAVE YOUR CAKE

372. ▪ **Dinner quick breads can double nicely as subtly sweet desserts.** This moist, feather-light zucchini bread succeeds in both roles. If you would like to dress it up for a sweeter dessert, serve it with Whipped Cream Frosting or Pineapple Frosting in tip 378 or 380. *Two Sweet Teeth.*

▪ ▪ ▪

▪ WHOLE-WHEAT ZUCCHINI BREAD* ▪

1½ cups whole-wheat flour
1 teaspoon baking soda
½ teaspoon salt
½ teaspoon each ground cinnamon and ground allspice
½ cup oil
¼ cup unsweetened apple-juice concentrate or
    pineapple-juice concentrate
1 egg plus 2 egg whites
3 tablespoons peach spreadable fruit
2 teaspoons natural vanilla extract
2 tablespoons water
1½ cups shredded zucchini (about 1 medium)

Preheat oven to 350 degrees. Lightly oil a 9-by-5-inch loaf pan and set aside. In a large bowl, mix together the dry ingredients. In a medium bowl, combine the liquid ingredients, then pour the liquids into the flour mixture and stir until just blended. Fold in the zucchini and pour into the loaf pan. Bake 45–55 minutes, or until a toothpick inserted in the center comes out clean. Cool on rack for 10 minutes; remove from pan and cool completely. *Makes 1 loaf or 12 servings.* ▪

373. ▪ **Whole-grain Belgian waffles for dessert?** You bet. They can substitute as easy fill-ins for shortcake when berries are in season and the idea of strawberry shortcake is beckoning. Van's makes a good line of frozen waffles you can heat up and use for such a purpose.

374. ▪ **What's carrot cake without the concentrated sweetening** of sugar, honey, or juice concentrate? Still very good

---

*This recipe was adapted from a Whole-Wheat Zucchini Bread that appeared in *The All-Natural Sugar-Free Dessert Cookbook* by Linda Romanelli Leahy.

when both moistness and varying textures are components of the cake. In this recipe from *Sweet and Natural*, Janet Warrington forgoes a concentrated sweetener of any kind and uses shredded carrot and bits of pineapple and raisins to give subtle bursts of sweetness in every bite. *One Sweet Tooth.*

▪ CARROT CAKE ▪

3 large carrots
1 large egg
$^3/_8$ cup oil
1 8-ounce can crushed pineapple, packed in its own juice
1 cup raisins
1 teaspoon natural vanilla extract
$1^1/_2$ cups whole-wheat flour
1 teaspoon ground cinnamon
$^1/_4$ teaspoon ground nutmeg
$^1/_4$ teaspoon ground allspice
$^1/_2$ teaspoon salt
$1^1/_2$ teaspoons baking powder

Scrub and grate the carrots. Measure 1 cup and set aside. Prepare an 8-inch-square baking pan with oil or a lecithin/oil combination. In a blender, combine egg, oil, crushed pineapple and juice, raisins, and vanilla. Process until raisins are finely chopped. Measure flour, spices, salt, and baking powder into a large mixing bowl. Stir well. Add blended mixture and grated carrots to dry ingredients, mixing until batter is uniform. Spread batter into oiled pan and bake at 350 degrees for 45–50 minutes or until cake tester comes out clean. Cool. Refrigerate. *Serves 8 to 10 people.* ▪

375. ▪ **Want to treat yourself to a rich piece of cake but don't have time to bake?** That's when individual thaw-and-serve portions of cakes by Amy's come in handy. Wholesome ingredients and no-fuss preparation—now that's my idea of pure indulgence! *Three Sweet Teeth.*

376. ▪ **Decadent chocolate desserts** are possible without refined sugar. This delicious recipe, courtesy of the Chatfield's company, will satisfy even the most confirmed chocolate lovers. *Three Sweet Teeth.*

▪ CATHERINE'S FAVORITE CHOCOLATE CAKE ▪

$1^2/_3$ cups whole-wheat flour
$^3/_4$ cup date "sugar"
$^1/_4$ cup unsweetened cocoa powder
1 teaspoon baking soda
$^1/_2$ teaspoon salt
1 cup water
$^1/_3$ cup oil
1 teaspoon vinegar
1 teaspoon natural vanilla extract

Heat oven to 350 degrees. Mix flour, date "sugar," cocoa powder, baking soda, and salt with a fork in an ungreased 8-inch baking dish. Mix in remaining ingredients. Bake until a wooden toothpick inserted in the center comes out clean, about 35–40 minutes. *Serves 8 to 10 people.* ▪

Note: You can also use Sucanat in place of date "sugar" in this recipe.

▪ ▪ ▪

ICING ON THE CAKE

377. ▪ **A frosting suitable even for most sugar-restricted diets** is Yogurt Cheese Icing suggested by Janet Warrington in her book *Sweet and Natural*. To make the icing, combine enough pureed fruit with Yogurt Cheese (from tip 106) to make a mixture that you can spread thinly over cake. *One Sweet Tooth.*

378. ▪ **Whipped Cream Frosting is dressy** despite being simple. Whether sweetened with honey, maple syrup, mashed banana, pureed fruit, or stevia powder—or even when it is used unsweetened—whipped cream works well on a wide variety of cakes. *One to Two Sweet Teeth.*

379. ▪ **Everyone is so concerned with the fat content of cream cheese frosting** that no one seems to realize that there's up to *a cup of sugar* in the typical cream-cheese-based icing. Nancy Burrows, author of *Allergy Cooking Tricks and Treasures,* suggests making a low-sugar version of this popular favorite by softening an 8-ounce package of cream cheese in a mixer with one of the following: 1–2 teaspoons honey or maple syrup; 1–2 tablespoons orange juice; 1–2 teaspoons honey and 1 table-spoon fresh lemon juice; *or* 1 teaspoon vanilla extract and 1 tea-spoon sweetener. If the mixture is too thick to spread the icing easily, add a few tablespoons of water or milk to create the con-sistency you want. *One to Two Sweet Teeth.*

380. ▪ **Here's a slightly sweeter version of cream-cheese frosting** that's particularly good on minimally sweetened cakes such as the Carrot Cake in tip 374. It comes from *Rodale's Basic Natural Foods Cookbook. Two Sweet Teeth.*

▪ ▪ ▪

▪ PINEAPPLE FROSTING ▪

3 ounces of cream cheese, softened
1 8-ounce can unsweetened, crushed pineapple, drained,
  with juice reserved
½ teaspoon natural vanilla extract
1 teaspoon honey

In a medium bowl, beat together the cream cheese, 2 table-spoons of the reserved pineapple juice, vanilla, and honey. Fold in crushed pineapple and refrigerate until it's thick enough to spread. *Makes 1 cup.* ▪

381. ▪ **Kozlowski Farms apple butter or fruit spread** can also be used as an instant way to frost cakes.

382. ▪ **Or create a quick nut-butter cake glaze.** Just add a little maple syrup or honey, vanilla extract, and/or carob powder to the nut butter, mix together, and spread.

383. ▪ **When a special occasion calls for a "splurge,"** try this versatile, easy-to-make frosting that's rich in flavor but still lower in sugars than most traditional frostings. It comes from *Kid Smart: Raising a Healthy Child* by Cheryl Townsley. *Three Sweet Teeth.*

▪ CAROB OR CHOCOLATE FROSTING ▪

¼ cup milk, almond milk, soy milk, or rice milk
¼ cup unsweetened carob or cocoa powder
2 tablespoons almond butter
3 to 4 tablespoons maple syrup
4 teaspoons arrowroot powder, or more as needed
¼ cup milk, almond milk, soy milk, or rice milk

Combine the first four ingredients in a blender and blend until smooth. Transfer to a small pan. Stir in arrowroot and remaining milk. Heat on low, stirring occasionally, until the mixture thickens to almost a frosting consistency (about 5 to 7 minutes), then remove from heat. It will thicken a little more as it cools. *Makes enough for one 9-inch-square cake.* ▪

384. ▪ **Instead of frosting a cake,** lightly dust one with coconut "sugar" (unsweetened shredded coconut finely ground in a blender).

385. ▪ **Or use powdered vanilla sugar,** a tasty topping you can make from recycled vanilla beans. After you've used vanilla beans, wipe them with a towel and allow them to dry on a plate overnight. Scrape away the little clumps of seeds from the pods and rub the clumps between your fingers to break them up. Add the seeds and plunge the pods into a jar of any dry sweetener—such as date "sugar," rice-syrup powder, or Sucanat—and allow the vanilla flavor and aroma to penetrate the sugar for four to five days. You can sprinkle vanilla sugar on top of cream cheese as a cake topping or, for special occasions, powder it in a blender to lightly dust cakes.

386. ▪ **If you think frosting is the only way you can decorate cakes,** think again. Scraped carrot twirls, nuts, or sliced fruit artfully arranged on top of cakes make delightfully attractive, low-sugar presentations. Other especially impressive decorations are pesticide-free, edible flowers such as brightly colored pansies, rose petals, marigolds, or nasturtiums.

PIES AND CRISPS

387. ▪ **There's no nicer way of enjoying the fruit in season** than making a fresh fruit pie. Unfortunately, most fruit pies are filled with *as much as a cup and a half of sweetener* in addition to all that delicious fruit. This recipe from Carol Nostrand's *Junk Food to Real Food* avoids all that added sugar, but you'll never miss it. Simply by soaking fresh apples and raisins in lemon juice and cinnamon, she has created an apple pie filling that ranks right up there with the best of them. *Two Sweet Teeth.*

▪ RAW FRUIT PIE WITH APPLE FILLING ▪

Crust

> 2 cups ground walnuts
> ¾ pound soft dried dates, pitted and chopped

Filling

> 3 large Golden Delicious apples, peeled, cored, quartered,
>   and sliced into ¼-inch-thick segments
> ³/₄ cup raisins
> Juice of 1½ small lemons (about 4 tablespoons)
> 1 teaspoon ground cinnamon

To make the crust, blend walnuts to a fine powder in a food processor or blender. Chop the dates in a food processor or blender. Then knead the crust ingredients together. Press into a 10-inch pie plate. Refrigerate overnight to help the crust harden. Also overnight soak the apples and raisins in the lemon juice and cinnamon. The next day spoon the filling into the pie crust and serve. *Makes one 10-inch pie. Serves 8–10 people.* ▪

388. ▪ **When converting your favorite pie recipes** using the tips in this book, start with the crust. Remember, refined white flour is out; whole grain is in. Here's a basic Whole-Wheat Crust that you can use in all your favorite recipes. It comes from *Sweet and Natural* by Janet Warrington.

▪ WHOLE-WHEAT CRUST ▪

1 cup whole-wheat flour
¼ teaspoon salt
¼ teaspoon oil
2 tablespoons ice water

In a medium bowl, fork-stir flour and salt to thoroughly mix. Combine oil and water in a measuring cup and pour it into the flour mixture. Stir until all ingredients are moistened. Pour the pastry mixture into a pie plate and flatten it across the bottom and up the sides of the plate using your fingers, the back of a spoon, or the outside of an empty measuring cup. Be careful to distribute the pastry evenly. For an empty shell, bake at 400 degrees for 15 minutes. *Makes enough for 1 whole pie.* ▪

389. ▪ **If you're in a hurry,** give yourself the luxury of using a wholesome frozen whole-wheat crust. Mother Nature's Goodies makes a good one you should be able to find in your local health-food store.

390. ▪ **Heat-and-serve frozen pies** are also available from Mother Nature's Goodies. They're a good alternative to most other store-bought pies, but still quite sweet. *Three Sweet Teeth.*

391. ▪ **Using a combination of fruit-flavored applesauce and fruit spread** as sweeteners produces flavorful desserts that are much lower in sugars than the same desserts sweetened with sugar, honey, or juice concentrate. This recipe is not quite a cobbler, but it is not your typical pie recipe either because it's much simpler. Mixing everything together instead of making a separate pie crust and pie filling saves time and effort. That's why it's "magic." *Two Sweet Teeth.*

▪ ▪ ▪

▪ MAGIC PEACH COBBLER PIE* ▪

1 cup brown-rice flour
1/4 to 1/2 teaspoon salt
1/4 teaspoon ground nutmeg
1 teaspoon ground cinnamon
1 teaspoon cream of tartar
4 cups fresh peaches, peeled and thinly sliced
1/3 cup oil
1/2 cup peach applesauce
3 tablespoons peach fruit spread
1 teaspoon almond extract
1 teaspoon baking soda
2 tablespoons boiling water

Oil and lightly dust with flour a 10-inch pie pan. Stir together the dry ingredients in a large bowl. Then preheat the oven to 350 degrees. Combine the oil, peach applesauce, fruit spread, and almond extract together, then add them to the flour mixture and mix well. Combine the baking soda and boiling water, stir to dissolve, and add to the batter. Quickly fold in the peaches, then scrape the batter into the pie pan and place in oven. Bake 40–50 minutes, or until pie is brown and peaches are tender. *Serves 8 to 10 people.* ▪

Note: To make a Magic Apple Cobbler Pie, substitute 1/2 cup applesauce, 3 tablespoons apple butter, and 4 cups of thinly sliced baking apples in place of the peach applesauce, peach fruit spread, and peaches. Delete the almond extract.

392. ▪ **Here's a Cherry Crisp recipe** that allows both the tartness and the sweetness of cherries to come through. It's

---

*This recipe was adapted from a recipe for Magic Apple Pie in *The Yeast Connection Cookbook* by William G. Crook, M.D., and Marjorie Hurt Jones, R.N.

quite a refreshing change from the usual sugar-laden cherry desserts. It's a creation of Deborah E. Buhr, author of *The "I Can't Believe This Has No Sugar" Cookbook. Two Sweet Teeth.*

■ CHERRY CRISP WITH DOUBLE-OAT TOPPING ■

Fruit Bottom

> 2 cups fresh or frozen, thawed, and drained dark sweet
>   cherries
> 2 tablespoons oil
> 3½ teaspoons tapioca
> ⅓ to ½ cup unsweetened pineapple-juice concentrate
> 2 tablespoons water

Topping

> ½ to ¾ cup rolled oats
> ¼ cup oat flour (or finely ground oats)
> 3 tablespoons oil
> 2 tablespoons sesame seeds
> ⅛ to ¼ teaspoon ground cinnamon

Stir all ingredients together except those for topping. Pour mixture into prepared baking dish and let sit for 10 minutes. Preheat oven to 350 degrees. Meanwhile, stir together Double-Oat Topping ingredients with a fork in a medium bowl. Spoon topping over cherry mixture and bake for 50 minutes. *Serves 6 to 8 people.* ■

393. ■ **Avoid store-bought cheesecake:** The main ingredient is cheap refined sugar. The following recipe for cheesecake is simple and requires no baking. Even more important, it's so luscious that you'll be amazed that it's sweetened with just fruit! *Two Sweet Teeth.*

▪ NO-BAKE PINEAPPLE CHEESECAKE* ▪

Crust

½ cup ground walnuts
½ cup pitted and ground dates
½ cup unsweetened shredded coconut
¼ teaspoon ground cinnamon

Filling

1 pound of light cream cheese, softened
½ cup nonfat yogurt
1 8-ounce can crushed pineapple, packed in its own juice,
   with juice reserved

Topping

¼ cup crushed or ground walnuts

Butter or oil a 9-inch pie plate. In a blender or food processor, grind the walnuts, transfer to a bowl, then grind the dates. Knead together all of the crust ingredients and press onto sides and bottom of the prepared pie plate. Put it into the refrigerator to chill. To make the filling, blend cream cheese in a large bowl until smooth. Fold in the yogurt and the reserved juice from the canned pineapple and mix well. Carefully add the crushed pineapple and stir just until blended. Spoon filling into the chilled pie crust and chill for several hours or overnight so flavors are well blended. Before serving, sprinkle crushed walnuts over top. *Makes one 9-inch cake. Serves 8 to 10 people.* ▪

*This recipe was adapted from a No-Bake Cheese Pie recipe in *Rodale's Basic Natural Foods Cookbook* by Charles Gerras, Editor, and the staff of Rodale Press.

SATISFYING COOKIES

394. ▪ **When I want to treat myself to a cookie,** the last thing I want is the fat-free kind—for two reasons. First, as a consumer who likes the taste of good food, I know I won't be satisfied with the fatless, sawdust-textured variety. Second, as a nutritionist who has studied the sugar issue for more than twenty years, I know that *fat-free* almost always means "more sugar than you bargained for." The key to healthy cookie enjoyment, I have found, is to treat yourself to one with *moderate* amounts of both sugar and fat—and hopefully some fiber as well.

395. ▪ **Chocolate chip** is the cookie of choice for most Americans when they want a treat. It's clear Americans are crazy about chocolate chips: 70 percent of the population actually keeps a package of semisweet chocolate morsels at home to bake with. The sugar-smart way to still enjoy chocolate chip cookies but get the sugar out of them is to use malt-sweetened chips such as those made by Sunspire or Chatfield's instead of the sugar-sweetened ones made by Nestlé or Hershey's.

396. ▪ **Adding high-fiber ingredients such as oats** to cookie recipes is a good way to slow down and lessen the body's response to the sugar in these sweets. This recipe from Melissa Diane Smith, for moist, scrumptious Oatmeal–Chocolate Chip Cookies, illustrates this concept well. *Two Sweet Teeth.*

▪ ▪ ▪

▪ OATMEAL–CHOCOLATE CHIP COOKIES ▪

1 cup raisins (golden raisins produce a lighter-color
   cookie)
1 cup unsweetened apple juice
¼ cup oil
1 cup oat flour *or* finely ground oats
1 cup oatmeal
½ teaspoon baking soda
¾ teaspoon ground cinnamon
¾ cup malt-sweetened chocolate chips
½ cup chopped walnuts (optional)

Soak the raisins in the juice overnight. The next day, puree
them together in a blender, then add the oil and blend again
briefly. Combine the rest of the ingredients in a mixing bowl,
making sure to mix well. Add the raisin-juice mixture and stir
just until mixed. Drop heaping teaspoonfuls of the batter onto
an ungreased baking sheet and bake at 375 degrees for 15–18
minutes, or until the cookies are lightly browned. *Makes about 3
dozen cookies.* ▪

397. ▪ **If you want to avoid the blood-sugar-raising caffeine in chocolate chips,** substitute malt-sweetened carob chips
in the above recipe. *Two Sweet Teeth.*

398. ▪ **If you're a macaroon fan,** try these cookies, which
combine the subtle sweetening power of brown-rice syrup powder, lemon extract, and grated lemon peel to produce delightfully light Lemony Almond Macaroon Drops. *One Sweet Tooth.*

▪ ▪ ▪

▪ LEMONY ALMOND MACAROON DROPS ▪

1 cup ground blanched almonds
3 egg whites
1 tablespoon lemon extract or natural vanilla extract
4½ tablespoons brown-rice syrup powder
1 tablespoon grated lemon peel
21 whole almonds

Mix together the ground blanched almonds, egg whites, flavoring extract, brown-rice syrup powder, and lemon peel. Mix until well blended, then chill the dough for one hour. Drop by heaping teaspoons onto an oiled cookie sheet. Press a whole almond into the top of each cookie and bake at 350 degrees until light brown, about 5 minutes. Cookies will harden more as they cool. *Makes 21 cookies.* ▪

399. ▪ **Naturally sweetened packaged cookies that taste like homemade** are available, and one of the best brands is a line called Pamela's. With varieties ranging from ginger cookies to butter shortbread to almond anise biscotti, Pamela's cookies are so wholesome that usually one cookie is all you need for total satisfaction. They're available in natural-food stores nationwide. *Two Sweet Teeth.*

400. ▪ **The sweetening power of plain mashed banana** continues to amaze me. Mashed banana is the only sweetener in these cookies, which are one of my staff members' favorites. *Two Sweet Teeth.*

▪ ▪ ▪

▪ CHEWY BANANA-OAT COOKIES* ▪

1½ cups oats
½ cup whole-wheat pastry flour, oat flour, *or* millet flour
½ teaspoon salt
¼ teaspoon baking soda
Dash or two of ground cinnamon (optional)
2 tablespoons chopped nuts or raisins
2 medium bananas, mashed (about 1 cup)
⅜ cup oil

Preheat oven to 350 degrees. Mix dry ingredients. In a separate bowl, mix mashed bananas and oil, then add to the dry ingredients. Drop by heaping teaspoons on an unoiled cookie sheet. Bake 10–15 minutes. *Makes about 2 dozen cookies.* ▪

Note: These cookies freeze well. You can double this recipe and freeze some for future treats.

401. ▪ **To make Oatmeal Harvest Cookies,** use 1 cup of mashed sweet potato or mashed acorn squash in place of the mashed banana. *One Sweet Tooth.*

▪ BONUS TIP: *You can also create other varieties of these whole-grain cookies by eliminating the oats and using rolled wheat flakes, barley flakes, rye flakes, spelt flakes, or kamut flakes instead.*

*This recipe was adapted from an Oatmeal Cookie recipe submitted by Ann Fisk, R.N., that appeared in the October 1988 issue of the *Mastering Food Allergies* newsletter.

▪ ▪ ▪

NATURAL CANDY

402. ▪ **Candy is a multibillion-dollar business** and one of the top three snack foods Americans consume. According to *Confectioner* magazine, just the U.S.-factory value of M&M's Chocolate Candies in 1994 alone was *more than $600 million.* It's important to remember that candy gives us lots of calories but little nutrition, yet manufacturers develop elaborate advertising campaigns and sponsorships to hook kids into the candy habit while they're still young and impressionable. Do your kids and yourself a favor by saying no to the heavily advertised, nutrient-poor commercial candies, and learn to satisfy your need for something sweet with the natural alternatives suggested in this section.

403. ▪ **Great substitutes for hard candy** are frozen grapes, raspberries, and blueberries. *One Sweet Tooth.*

404. ▪ **So are dried fruits,** which are nature's concentrated sources of natural sugars as well as vitamins, minerals, and fiber. *Three Sweet Teeth.*

▪ BONUS TIP: *It's worth it to seek out unsulfured dried fruits for treats. Commercial dried fruits treated with sulfur dioxide can produce unpleasant symptoms such as nausea, headaches, and rashes, and sometimes even more serious, life-threatening allergic reactions.*

405. ▪ **When a bite of *rich* candy is what you want,** stuffed dates can naturally fulfill your wishes. Just pit a few dates and fill them with unsweetened peanut butter, almond butter, or cashew butter. You'll be surprised at how rich and filling these easy-to-make creations are. *Two Sweet Teeth.*

406. ▪ **Here's another convincing example** of how fruit can be candy. *Two Sweet Teeth.*

▪ FRUIT CANDY ▪

$\frac{1}{2}$ cup sesame seeds or chopped nuts
$\frac{1}{2}$ cup finely chopped dried fruit
$\frac{1}{4}$ teaspoon ground cinnamon or more to taste
1 cup unsweetened nut butter *or* seed butter
$\frac{1}{2}$ cup unsweetened shredded coconut

Lightly toast sesame seeds or chopped nuts in a 275-degree oven for a few minutes until they're fragrant and golden brown, being careful not to burn them. Stir the seeds or chopped nuts, chopped dried fruit, and cinnamon together in a medium-size bowl. Gradually add nut or seed butter, using just enough to form a soft dough. Roll dough into small ball or log shapes, then gently roll each of them in shredded coconut. Place on a cookie sheet or platter and refrigerate until serving. *Makes 2 to 3 dozen.* ▪

407. ▪ **Other ingredients to experiment with** when making no-bake dried-fruit candies are other nut butters or tahini; powdered grain-based coffee substitutes; vanilla, orange, or almond extracts; and peppermint, spearmint, or wintergreen oils.

408. ▪ **Carob powder and dry milk powder** are naturals in candy concoctions because they're both naturally sweet. This simple recipe is from *Sweet and Natural* by Janet Warrington. *Two Sweet Teeth.*

▪ ▪ ▪

▪ PEANUT BUTTER–CAROB BALLS ▪

1 cup natural-style peanut butter, smooth or crunchy
²⁄₃ cup packed, chopped raisins
3 tablespoons nonfat dry-milk powder
2 tablespoons carob powder
pinch salt (optional)
½ cup unsweetened shredded coconut (optional)

Combine all ingredients, except the coconut, in a large bowl. Shape into approximately 32 balls, rolling about 1 teaspoon dough between palms for each. If desired, roll the balls in coconut. Refrigerate in an airtight container or individually wrapped. ▪

409. ▪ **In the mood for chocolate?** That could be because chocolate supplies b-phenethylamine, the same chemical your brain produces when you're in love. Fortunately, a bite or two of chocolate is usually all that you need for a treat. A small piece provides that same luscious feel in your mouth that a large piece does, and a mini-"splurge" can be so satisfying that it can act as a natural deterrent against overindulging.

410. ▪ **If you're going to treat yourself to chocolate,** make sure you treat yourself to a naturally sweetened variety instead of the usual candy bar made with refined sugar. Try splitting a Chatfield's Truffle Bar with a friend or look for miniature individual chocolate squares (called changemakers) made by Tropical Source, a division of Cloud Nine, Inc. *Two Sweet Teeth.*

▪ ▪ ▪

GELATINS AND PUDDINGS

411. ▪ **J-E-L-L-O is nutrient-void S-U-G-A-R** no matter how you look at it. If you or your kids are fond of this common American dessert, make it the healthier way with unsweetened fruit juice. Just add 1 tablespoon unflavored gelatin to 2 cups of any kind of warm, unsweetened fruit juice. Stir until gelatin dissolves, then pour gelatin mixture into serving cups and chill until set. *Three Sweet Teeth.*

▪ BONUS TIP: *If you make gelatin fruit salad, do not add fresh pineapple, papaya, guava, kiwi, figs, or gingerroot to the gelatin. These foods contain enzymes that prevent the gelatin from setting.*

412. ▪ **Another healthier gelatin** can be made with agar-agar, a seaweed gelatin, in place of animal gelatin. Combine 2 cups unsweetened juice and 2 tablespoons agar-agar flakes in a saucepan and boil for 30 seconds. Cool for 20 minutes, then refrigerate until gelled. *Three Sweet Teeth.*

413. ▪ **Whipping up this pudding is a dream** because it's so ridiculously simple to make but it is amazingly sweet, rich, and creamy even though it's only sweetened with banana. It's another recipe from *Sweet and Natural* by Janet Warrington. *One Sweet Tooth.*

▪ PEANUT BUTTER PUDDING ▪

1 small, ripe banana
$\frac{1}{2}$ cup plain, nonfat yogurt
$\frac{1}{2}$ cup peanut butter, natural style
$\frac{1}{4}$ teaspoon natural vanilla extract
pinch salt (optional)

Combine all ingredients in a blender. Process on low, then high speed until smooth. Pour into 4 individual serving dishes and refrigerate. Serve cold. *Serves 4.* ▪

414. ▪ **Here's another blended dessert** that is a good substitute for sugar-sweetened, fruit-flavored yogurt. It was developed especially for this book by Holly Sollars, a former demonstration chef at Canyon Ranch health resort. *Two Sweet Teeth.*

▪ FRUITY TOFU DELIGHT ▪

1 10.5-ounce package of Mori-Nu extrafirm silken tofu
1½ cups unsweetened frozen cherries or other frozen
    fruit
4 tablespoons Kozlowski Farms cherry spread or other
    flavor all-fruit spread

Place tofu in a blender on medium until smooth and silky, stopping occasionally to scrape unblended tofu from the sides of the blender container. Add frozen fruit and process, then add fruit spread and blend until smooth. Serve immediately, or chill for several hours for a firmer consistency. *Makes 2 to 3 servings.* ▪

415. ▪ **Another quick pudding** can be made by blending about a pound of drained tofu, a 16-ounce can of drained pineapple, and honey and vanilla to taste. *Two Sweet Teeth.*

416. ▪ **Tapioca pudding is terrific,** especially when you replace the sugar in your favorite recipe with date "sugar," brown-rice syrup powder, rice syrup, barley malt, honey, or maple syrup. *Two Sweet Teeth.*

417. ▪ **Bread pudding is another recipe that's easy to adapt.** Use a natural sweetener in place of sugar and be sure to use whole-grain-bread cubes instead of white-bread cubes. *Two Sweet Teeth.*

418. ▪ **Rice pudding is delicious** made with short-grain brown rice instead of white rice. (I think it's better.) I also like it because it's an easy way to use up leftover brown rice you have in the refrigerator and because you can make it in a variety of ways—in the Crock-Pot, in a saucepan on the stovetop, or baked in the oven. This recipe, from *Smart Breakfasts* by Jane Kinderlehrer, is a way to bake Brown Rice Pudding in the oven. *Two Sweet Teeth.*

▪ BROWN RICE PUDDING ▪

2 eggs
2 cups milk (2% milk makes a creamier pudding than
    nonfat does)
¼ cup honey or rice syrup
1 teaspoon natural vanilla extract
1½ cups cooked short-grain brown rice
½ cup raisins
dash of grated nutmeg and/or ground cinnamon

Preheat oven to 350 degrees. In a food processor or mixing bowl, blend together the eggs, milk, sweetener, and vanilla. Stir in the brown rice and raisins. Spoon into a 1-quart casserole and dust with nutmeg and/or cinnamon. Bake for 1 to 1½ hours. Pudding is done when a knife inserted in the center comes out clean. Serve hot with milk or cream, or chill and serve plain. *Serves 8.* ▪

▪ ▪ ▪

FROZEN TREATS

419. ▪ **The light, refreshing sweetness of frozen pureed fruit** comes through whether you make it into a sorbet or a Popsicle. To make sorbet for four people, place about 2 cups of pureed fruit combined with 1 teaspoon of honey or a pinch of fructose in a plastic container and freeze for 2 hours. Take out and stir well, then return to the freezer to freeze completely. Allow it to sit for 15 minutes at room temperature before serving. Any kind of fruit works in this recipe, but sorbet made out of cantaloupe, mango, grapefruit, or berries seems particularly refreshing to me on hot summer days. *Two Sweet Teeth.*

420. ▪ **To make a popsicle out of pureed fruit,** Carol Nostrand, author of *Junk Food to Real Food,* suggests blending sliced fresh fruit (about 1½ fruit servings per person) with a little bit of water and pouring the fruit puree into Popsicle molds or leftover small juice-concentrate cans. Put Popsicle sticks in the mold, then allow the mold to freeze until solid. To serve, run warm water over the outside of the can and the popsicle will slip out. *Two Sweet Teeth.*

421. ▪ **Or make fruit Creamsicles.** Follow the instructions above except use one piece of blended fruit (for example, one chopped medium peach) blended with 3–4 tablespoons low-fat yogurt and ¼ teaspoon natural vanilla extract. *Two Sweet Teeth.*

422. ▪ **What tastes like frozen custard on the inside** and nutty Swiss almond ice cream on the outside? "Gone Nutty" Frozen Bananas—a perfect cool treat on a sticky summer afternoon. *Two Sweet Teeth.*

▪ ▪ ▪

▪ "GONE NUTTY" FROZEN BANANAS ▪

¼ cup almond milk
3 tablespoons almond butter
¼ teaspoon almond extract
2 ripe bananas
½ cup lightly toasted ground almonds

Blend together the almond milk, almond butter, and almond extract in a blender. Peel the bananas, cut them in half, and roll them in the almond liquid coating, then roll them in the lightly toasted ground almonds. Place on a small plate and freeze until solid. Allow to thaw for at least 15 minutes before eating. *Serves 4.* ▪

423. ▪ **What's ice cream without refined sugar?** Very good, and it's possible to make it even if you don't have an ice cream machine. In this recipe, Nancy Burrows, author of *Allergy Cooking Tricks and Treasures*, shows us how. *Three Sweet Teeth.*

▪ VANILLA ICE CREAM ▪

1 teaspoon gelatin
2 tablespoons cold water
1 12-ounce can of unsweetened evaporated milk
⅓ cup honey or maple syrup
2 teaspoons nautral vanilla extract

Sprinkle gelatin over cold water in standard mixing bowl. Let soften 10 minutes. Heat half of milk to very hot or scalding. (A double boiler prevents burning.) Add hot milk to gelatin mixture and stir to dissolve. Add remaining milk. Chill. (The freezer speeds up this step.) Whip cold mixture with electric mixer until soft peaks form, about 8–10 minutes. Add sweetener and vanilla and mix to incorporate thoroughly. Freeze in covered container. *Makes about 1¾ quarts.* ▪

Note: You can make mint ice cream by adding one drop of real peppermint extract to the above recipe. *Three Sweet Teeth.*

424. ▪ **Chocolate ice cream without milk and sugar?** Sure, it's easy when pureed bananas serve as the combination creamy base and sweetener. This delectable recipe comes from *The "I Can't Believe This Has No Sugar" Cookbook* by Deborah E. Buhr. *Three Sweet Teeth.*

▪ CHOCOLATE ICE CREAM ▪

4 bananas, peeled
4 squares Baker's All-Natural Unsweetened Chocolate
3 tablespoons water

In a medium-sized bowl, mash the bananas. Melt chocolate with water in the top of a double boiler. Add melted chocolate and water to bananas, stir, and freeze before serving. *Makes 4 servings.* ▪

CHAPTER 8

Get the Sugar Out
When You Eat Out

There is perhaps no greater challenge to reducing the sugar in your diet than getting the sugar out when you eat out. After all, when you decide to give yourself a break from cooking and let others cook for you instead, you give up some control in exchange for convenience (and perhaps also for ambience, sociability, and just plain pampering). You no longer choose every ingredient or how much of every ingredient is put into the food you are served. Hidden sugar can thus sneak into your food unless you develop the know-how to keep the sugar out.

A big part of keeping the sugar out when you eat out is knowing what to expect from the average eatery. For example, if you order pancakes at a typical restaurant, you should obviously not expect to be served whole-grain cakes and pure maple syrup. Similarly, if you order rice off a menu, it will be white rice; pasta off a menu will be white pasta; and bread off a menu will be white bread unless the menu specifically tells you otherwise. In addition, desserts will almost always be made with white flour and white sugar—the kinds we should all avoid—unless you go out of your way to get one at a natural-food restaurant. The trick to avoiding these nutrient-

poor carbohydrates when dining out, then, is either to frequent restaurants that offer whole-grain choices on the menu
(something I try to do when I'm traveling) or to dine at other
restaurants and just skip the processed starches as much as
possible and emphasize more vegetables.

If you're like many people today, you may eat out more
often than you eat in. Once you have an idea of what to expect
when eating out, it is much easier to know what and how to
order to avoid unwanted sugars. Knowing how to get low-sugar
foods—whether at a fast-food chain, a Chinese restaurant, or a
four-star gourmet restaurant—is a basic survival skill that all of
us need to learn.

The tips in this chapter cover this important topic as well as
the equally important subject of what foods you should take on
short excursions and long trips. These tips will teach you how to
eat nutritiously on the run so you can keep up a healthful pace.

GETTING WHAT YOU WANT

425. ▪ **Don't be afraid to ask questions** like "What's in
that?" or "How is that prepared?" Remember that your waiter
or waitress is at the restaurant to serve you. It's in the restaurant's best interests to have a satisfied customer, so don't feel
sheepish about politely making special requests, particularly
when your emotional and physical health depend upon it.

426. ▪ **Pick and choose from the menu.** If a food is on the
menu, you should be able to get it, even though it may not be
listed with the particular entrée you want. A grilled chicken
breast, for example, may be topped with a sugar-rich barbecue
sauce, while a pasta dish (made from white flour) might be

teamed with a fresh tomato-and-basil marinara sauce. You should be able to combine the best aspects of the two entrées and get a chicken breast topped with the marinara sauce—an entrée that eliminates sugars and refined carbohydrates completely.

427. ▪ **One of the toughest challenges** when eating in restaurants today is avoiding processed carbohydrates such as white rice, pasta, and bread. It's easiest just to skip the starches and ask for a double order of veggies or salad instead.

428. ▪ **Be clear about what you want** and stress to your servers that you are following a diet in which you need to avoid sugar and other sweeteners. Restaurant servers are more likely to pay attention when you tell them that you *need* to avoid sugar instead of that you want to. (It should not matter whether you are eliminating sugar because of a yeast infection, heart disease, hypoglycemia, or just to feel your best. The restaurant should take your desire to avoid sugar as seriously as it does a diabetic's.)

429. ▪ **Ask for a particularly accommodating server by name** when making reservations at a restaurant you frequent. If you've gotten the kind of food and service you've wanted from that server before, you can expect to get it again. It's nice to have established a close enough relationship with your server to say, "I'll have the usual," and know that he or she will get your order right, no questions asked.

▪ BONUS TIP: *Be sure to reward your special server (or any accommodating server) with both praise and a generous tip. These will go a long way toward ensuring that you get the same quality service in the future.*

430. ▪ **Natural-food restaurants are worth seeking out.** When you find one, you can be assured that the selections offered are made with fresh, wholesome ingredients. As a result, your meal is much less apt to contain hidden sugars. In addition, eating at a natural-food restaurant often means you can treat yourself to tasty whole-grain dishes and naturally sweetened desserts that are simply not available at other restaurants.

MENU SAVVY

431. ▪ **Avoid the after-breakfast sugar blues** by steering clear of these typical sugar-rich restaurant breakfast foods: pastries, croissants, and muffins; white toast, bagels, English muffins, and fruit jam; pancakes, waffles, and all of their accompaniments; fruit crepes; granola and other sweetened cereals; fruit-flavored yogurt; and ham, bacon, and sausage.

432. ▪ **Don't be fooled into thinking "heart healthy" symbols** on a restaurant menu necessarily mean "blood sugar healthy." In fact, as more and more restaurant chefs try to reduce the fat in the meals they prepare, they are increasingly using sugar-rich glazes, marinades, and sauces. A sugar-laden pineapple-teriyaki-glazed chicken breast may qualify for a little heart symbol on a menu, but it's not an entrée for balancing blood-sugar levels. (We now know that it's not exactly heart healthy either because too much sugar contributes to heart problems.)

433. ▪ **Watch out for key menu words and phrases** that signal too much sugar. Anytime a food is served with a sweet glaze, syrup, or demiglacé, steer clear of it.

434. ▪ *Caramelized* is another term that usually means "sugarized."

435. ▪ **Avoid entrées that say they are served with the restaurant's "own special sweet sauce."** The main ingredient in many sweet sauces is usually refined sugar.

436. ▪ **The same is often true of barbecue sauces and honey-based mustards and salad dressings.** Pass up these disguised sugar sources whenever possible.

437. ▪ **Fruit sauces on entrées may sound healthy,** but they are apt to have a lot of empty-calorie sugar and wine in them and not much fruit. In general, ask that entrées be prepared without sugary sauces or at least ask for the sauce "on the side."

438. ▪ **The safest salad dressing to order** as far as sugar is concerned is vinegar and oil or lemon wedges and oil. Creamy commercial dressings that restaurants buy in bulk are common sources of hidden sugars.

▪ BONUS TIP: *With the help of two-ounce, watertight Tupperware containers known as Midgets, you can unobtrusively carry sugar-free dressings or unrefined oils with you just about anywhere you go.*

439. ▪ **Limit ordering so-called "light fare"** such as pasta salad or fruit salad served with sherbet or frozen yogurt. Remember that these foods are light on nutrition and heavy on nutrient-poor sugars and processed carbohydrates.

440. ▪ **Don't forget that one glass of soda or juice** gives you more sugar than most of us should consume in a single day. Order instead bottled water, mineral water, soda water, or iced or hot teas.

441. ▪ **Avoid ordering desserts in restaurants,** where you can't control the amount and type of sweeteners put in them. If you don't want to seem antisocial, try inviting your dining companions to your house for a healthier dessert.

442. ▪ **Or order a bowl of berries or a fruit salad,** which are the safest choices at the restaurant. Even if you do not see fruit on the menu, don't hesitate to ask for it. Most good restaurants have fruit in the kitchen to use in other desserts or for garnishes. They usually are more than willing to serve it to you.

INTERNATIONAL INSIGHTS

443. ▪ **Foreign cuisines not only offer variety,** they can also offer healthy, low-sugar eating as long as you use sugar savvy when ordering. Not all ethnic food is low in sugar, but it is often more healthful and less processed than American fare, particularly dishes where lots of fresh vegetables are emphasized.

444. ▪ **If you decide to go Italian** (as I often do), try not to make refined pasta and refined bread the cornerstones of your meal. Choose instead deliciously prepared veal, chicken, fish, or shellfish with garlic and fresh herbs, and add a leafy green Italian salad and a medley of flavorful sautéed vegetables.

445. ▪ **When you want to eat Greek,** keep a few guidelines in mind: Avoid the Greek pastries; limit your intake of refined pasta, rice, and pita bread; and avoid dishes with honey-based sauces. Some good sugar-free Greek dishes to try include souvlaki, roast leg of lamb, chicken Athenian, shrimp Scorpios, and traditional Greek salad. *Avgolemono* soup (Greek egg-lemon soup) is particularly delicious and tastes sweet even though it contains no sugar.

446. ▪ **Chinese restaurants provide ample selections from which to choose** as long as you avoid sugar-containing sweet-and-sour, plum, and *hoisin* sauces. Request that no sugar be added to your meal during cooking. If your meal seems a little bland without any extra sugar, ask for hot mustard, minced garlic, scallions, or some Chinese five-spice powder from the kitchen to give your dish a little extra seasoning. Chinese five-spice powder is my particular favorite for sweetening a stir-fry without sugar.

447. ▪ **Japanese restaurants and Japanese steak houses** can not only provide healthful food, but also fun entertainment if they cook the food right at your table. When ordering, remember that any hibachi-style dish should be sugar-free, but not necessarily sukiyaki and teriyaki dishes. These are better avoided.

■ BONUS TIP: *Sushi is an increasingly popular offering at many Japanese restaurants. Although raw-fish-based sushi does not contain sugar, I do not recommend it because of the increasing amounts of parasites and contaminants found in seafood. To enjoy sushi from time to time, choose safe kinds made with avocado, cucumber, or cooked crab or shrimp.*

448. ■ **When the restaurant you visit is French,** stay away from the French pastries and sweet dishes such as duck *à l'orange*. Especially healthy French selections include fish *en papillote* (fish cooked in its own juices with herbs), poached salmon, *poulet aux fines herbes* (roast chicken with herbs), bouillabaisse, ratatouille, and salad niçoise.

449. ■ **In the mood for Mexican food?** Go ahead and enjoy it. Although some fast-food Mexican restaurants may add sugar to the food they serve, most good Mexican restaurants will not, so the main thing you have to avoid is tortillas made from refined flour. Opt for corn tortillas instead unless you're lucky enough to find a Mexican eatery or health-food restaurant that uses whole-wheat tortillas. Good selections to order at Mexican restaurants include gazpacho, beef tostadas, chicken or beef fajitas, bean burritos, and taco salad.

450. ■ **Indian dishes sometimes contain small amounts of naturally occurring sweet foods** such as raisins, but the amounts are usually small enough and balanced with enough protein and fat that they don't cause much of a blood-sugar problem. Such dishes as chicken and lamb tandoori, *korma*, or curry can all fit nicely into a low-sugar way of life, and basmati-rice-based *biryanis* or bean-based dals are good sources of healthful, unrefined complex carbohydrates.

ON THE RUN AND ON THE ROAD

451. ▪ **Limit your intake of typical fast food** because although it may be fast, most of it is a disaster for anyone trying to avoid sugar, salt, and nonessential fat. French fries at fast-food outlets frequently are dipped in a sugar solution before frying, beef patties may have sugar added to them as a flavor enhancer, and breadings for fried chicken and fish usually are sugar rich. Condiments such as ketchup, salad dressings, and "special sauces" aren't so special anymore when you realize that their key ingredient is most often sugar. The worst thing about fast food is that the more we eat it, the more we come to expect large amounts of sugar and salt in all of the foods we eat.

452. ▪ **Look for the increasingly popular fast-food outlets** that offer more healthful rotisserie-cooked chicken, turkey, and other home-style meals. Wholesome, low-sugar side dishes are also usually available at these eateries. Good choices to go with chicken and turkey include steamed, stewed, or baked vegetables, side salads, baked or mashed potatoes, roasted red potatoes, and sometimes even cooked sweet potatoes.

453. ▪ **Salad bars and a variety of prepackaged salads** are being offered at a number of outlets, including some of the bigger fast-food hamburger chains. If you know your schedule necessitates your picking up a salad to go, take along your own dressing (as described in bonus tip 438) to avoid the sugar-rich processed varieties.

454. ▪ **If for lunch you long for the food you eat at home,** invest in a widemouthed thermos and take food from home with you. Sugar-free soups and leftovers work particularly well in a thermos, and they make for inexpensive lunches. It's also comforting to eat your favorite foods even when you're away from home.

455. ▪ **A thermos also works well for making hot breakfast cereals** you can take with you in the morning or for making grain side dishes for trips and picnics. To make one serving of thermos cereal, follow these instructions from the authors of *Eating for A's:* Pour in ⅓ cup of hot water and 2 tablespoons of cracked wheat, couscous, bulgur wheat, or hot-water-soaked brown rice. Tighten the lid of the thermos and let stand anywhere from half an hour to five hours. Add herbs, spices, milk, nuts, or fruit if desired, or eat as is from the container.

456. ▪ **Meals-in-a-muffin,** explained earlier in tips 272 and 304, are the ultimate sugar-free fast food.

457. ▪ **So are balanced whole-food bars,** such as Balance bars made by BioFoods. Even though these bars contain a number of sugars, the sugars are balanced with high-quality protein and fat, and the whole bar registers only 36 percent on the Glycemic Index. The result is a convenient fast food that even many diabetics and hypoglycemics can use. (One bar equals one protein exchange and two fruit exchanges on the diabetic exchange system.) If you can't find Balance bars in your local health-food store, call 1-800-678-4246 to order them direct.

458. ▪ **When traveling by car,** pack some sugar-free snacks from home to avoid grabbing sugary snacks on the run. Peanut butter sandwiches, low-sugar granola bars, or nut-based trail mixes are three good choices. Review the tips in chapter 5 for other ideas.

459. ▪ **If you're traveling by plane, order a special meal** such as "diabetic," "lactovegetarian," "vegetarian," or "cold seafood plate." A special meal does not guarantee that everything on your plate will be sugar-free, but it is usually a tremendous improvement over the standard meals. Place your order when you reserve your ticket, and be sure to double-check on your special meal a day before your departure.

460. ▪ **Also take high-quality snacks with you on the plane** in case the airline makes a mistake or gives you something that is more sugary than you are expecting. High-protein snacks such as Balance bars (tip 457) or muffins made out of "supergrains" are better for traveling than the honey-roasted nuts, muffins, or other sugary bites that airlines typically serve. I usually find snacks from home much more satisfying than airline food anyway. For the sugar-free hydration that is desperately needed when flying, I also like to take along bottled water.

CHAPTER 9

Get the Sugar Out
of Your Mind and
Out of Your Life

I f you get the sugar out of your diet but continue to think about it every day and dream about it every night, the chances are not good that it will stay out of your diet for long.

That's because your beliefs, thoughts, and feelings really do have a huge impact on your actions. Current research into mind-body medicine shows that your thoughts even influence how your body physically perceives an experience. This means that if you work on altering your attitudes concerning sugar, your dietary transition away from sugar will be an easier and more successful one.

My experience with my clients seems to confirm the truth in these findings. Thinking back over the more than nine thousand clients I have seen, I can tell you that those individuals who have made the most positive and lasting dietary changes were the ones who made life-changing attitudinal transformations as well.

Of course, changing misconceived ideas is only one part of what is required to change long-standing eating habits. Other important parts are purely practical in nature—how you can get started, how you can stay motivated, and how you can cope with the physical, emotional, and social pressures that hold you back from changing.

This chapter covers these neglected but exceedingly important aspects to getting the sugar out. The tips include a potpourri of information, but this information can sometimes make all the difference in helping you stick to an eating plan that keeps the sugar out.

Eating so as to keep the sugar out over the long term is the only way to maintain your best weight, and it is far better than going on and off nutritionally unsound fad diets. Tips to remind you of this—and tips that cover the importance of regular exercise—are also included in this chapter.

A decision to keep the sugar out of your life is a commitment to health that must last a lifetime. The tips that follow will help you keep this important commitment so your efforts will pay off in sweet rewards.

GETTING STARTED

461. ▪ **Eliminate first the sugars that you are the least apt to miss:** those sugars that are hidden in drinks and in breakfast, lunch, and dinner convenience foods.

462. ▪ **Consult your doctor regularly** if you are currently taking medication. If you cut the sugar in your diet in a noticeable way, your cholesterol levels, blood pressure, or blood-sugar levels may change so dramatically that your medication may need to be reduced or perhaps eventually eliminated.

463. ▪ **Keep a food diary.** Jotting down everything you eat and drink for a few days is a sure-fire way of seeing the truth of your eating habits more clearly. Be sure to keep a record of what you eat on at least one weekend day, too, because we may eat irregularly and indulge in foods then that we don't usually have the rest of the week.

464. ▪ **Look for patterns in your food record,** in particular, when you crave and indulge in sweets. Several clients of mine who ate well the rest of the week were shocked at their sugar-craving mayhem on the weekends. Every weekend they went out for an unusually high-sugar breakfast: pancakes (made from white flour), high-sugar commercial pancake syrup, and a large glass of orange juice. This started a cycle that led to blood-sugar swings and sugar cravings and binges on those days.

465. ▪ **Make a bet to stay sugar-free.** You'd be amazed how sheer stubbornness and the desire to show the other person you can win the bet often give you unfailing resolve. (The opportunity to earn a little money doesn't hurt either.) A thirty-year-old career woman I know made a bet with her boss to give up chocolate for Lent. She had a difficult time not giving in to her desire for chocolate, but did it just to show him she could. The great thing was, after she won the bet, she felt so good, she decided not to go back to chocolate and to cut down on other forms of sugar as well!

466. ▪ **Try staying sugar-free Vegas style.** Find others who are trying to kick the sugar habit and encourage each person to bet money that both they and you can stick to a healthier, low-sugar lifestyle. If someone drops out, the rest of you get to split their money. Set the parameters so everyone clearly understands, and you'll be surprised by how well monetary bets keep you committed to getting the sugar out.

▪ ▪ ▪

EMOTIONAL CONSIDERATIONS

467. ▪ **Do not use sugar as a quick fix to help you "cope"** with stress and tension. This is a common mistake. Eating sugar actually backfires: It depletes nutrient reserves, taxes the endocrine glands, and actually causes the body more stress, making you feel worse than you did before.

468. ▪ **If you think sugar could not possibly have an effect on behavior,** consider this: The brain controls our behavior, thought process, memory, learning, and moods. It is affected by any sudden changes in blood sugar because it uses almost half of all the available sugar in the blood. Studies have shown that excess sugar intake by children increases their likelihood of antisocial behavior, anxiety, lack of concentration, irritability, and emotional outbursts.

469. ▪ **Be aware of the emotional factors** behind when you desire sugar. See if you can make any connections between when you most want sugar and what types of things you are feeling then. If you find that you want sugar when you are most upset, talk to a trusted friend, meditate, take a relaxing bath, or try other ways to feel better that don't involve food.

470. ▪ **Don't fall into the trap of believing sugar will make you happy.** The pleasure you may experience from sugar on your taste buds is just temporary. It doesn't change any unhappiness you may be feeling from troubles with your friends, family, work, or love. Remember, too, that sugar often causes depression and emotional upset, besides being a major contributor to the development of physical diseases that can affect us emotionally.

▪ ▪ ▪

NUTRIENT NECESSITIES

471. ▪ **Chromium, manganese, and zinc,** three trace minerals in short supply in the average American's diet, are needed to control blood-sugar levels. Individuals with consistently low levels of these minerals are often diabetic. If you have hypoglycemia, diabetes, or any type of blood-sugar trouble, supplementation with these minerals is advisable. The usual daily dose is 200 to 600 micrograms of chromium, 10 to 30 milligrams of manganese, and 30 to 50 milligrams of zinc. Be sure the supplements you take are free of sugar.

472. ▪ **If you have intense cravings for sugar,** try taking 500 milligrams of the brain-feeding nutrient l-glutamine, up to three times per day. In the brain, l-glutamine converts to glutamic acid, the only source of glucose besides sugar that the brain can use for energy. This amino acid is extremely helpful for people with hypoglycemia, and it has worked wonders for some of my most sugar-craving clients.

473. ▪ **Support your adrenal glands for better blood-sugar balance.** The adrenals are constantly at work helping your body cope with such stresses as going too long without food or too much sugar. Since they are so important to blood sugar and health in general, be sure to nourish the adrenal glands with the vitamins and minerals they need—nutrients such as B-complex vitamins, pantothenic acid, vitamin C, zinc, and manganese. If you are stressed and your blood sugar is unbalanced, you might also want to consider taking adrenal and pancreatic glandular bovine tissue. With their RNA-DNA blueprints so similar to our own, these glandulars have proven extremely helpful for strengthening the adrenal and pancreatic function of many of my clients.

474. ▪ **No matter how many nutrients you take,** remember that sugar is an antinutrient that literally throws most of those nutrients down the toilet. Sugar is known to interfere with the absorption, or to increase the excretion, of the B vitamins and almost all minerals. Your body requires large amounts of these nutrients to digest and assimilate nutrients from all the foods you eat. The best thing you can do to improve your nutrient status is not to take more supplements but to eat less sugar!

475. ▪ **This is especially true for your calcium and magnesium levels.** Both calcium and magnesium are excreted in the urine after sugar ingestion. No matter how much of these minerals you take in food and supplemental form, if you take them with a lot of sugar, you will not be able to absorb them. Since these minerals are crucial for strong bones, the huge rise in sugar intake may, in fact, be the primary reason for the high incidence of osteoporosis in the United States today.

THE ACTIVE INGREDIENT

476. ▪ **If your discipline momentarily breaks down** and you eat some type of sweet concoction, don't despair. There's a simple solution: Walk, run, take a bike ride, play some tennis. Exercise in whatever way you like best so your body can use that sugar for energy instead of fat storage.

477. ▪ **Make social times active times.** Plan gatherings not around eating sugar but around exercise. For example, instead of meeting for coffee and dessert, schedule a tennis match or power walk or go out dancing.

478. ▪ **Why exercise regularly?** Because it's one of the most beneficial things you can do for your blood sugar and for your health. Regular exercise can lower blood-sugar levels in diabetics and make insulin more effective for muscle and fat cells. It can also improve the body's absorption of nutrients, help prevent heart disease and osteoporosis, and increase the body's resistance to disease. In addition, regular exercise plays a key role in helping us look and feel our best. It helps create a feeling of emotional well-being, relieving irritability, anxiety, and depression. Physically, it increases the body's endurance, muscle strength, and flexibility, and it promotes weight loss and weight control.

479. ▪ **You do not have to be a marathon runner to get the benefits of exercise.** Even a brisk twenty-minute walk four or more times a week will do. It does not matter so much at what level you start so long as you keep it up and gradually improve. Consistency is the key to receiving exercise's benefits.

480. ▪ **A little bit of a high-glycemic food** can give you a quick burst of energy for exercising, but don't use exercise as an excuse to overeat sugary foods. Too much sugar can even lessen the many beneficial effects of exercise.

SLIM FOR KEEPS

481. ▪ **Say no thanks to the latest unbalanced fad diet.** Starving yourself and living off grapefruit or sugar-rich "diet shakes" is not sensible, and the body knows it. A plan such as this may be a quick way to lose water weight and muscle mass, but it will do nothing for what you really want to lose—body fat. A fad starvation plan is also one of the quickest ways I know of to develop blood-sugar problems and a slower body metabolism, both of which will almost certainly lead to more weight gain, not weight loss.

482. ▪ **Diet foods sweetened with aspartame are diet no-no's.** As already mentioned in tip 53, ingestion of aspartame (also known as NutraSweet or Equal) suppresses production of serotonin, a neurotransmitter that controls eating patterns. Without adequate serotonin, the body experiences intense sugar and carbohydrate cravings, which can lead to uncontrollable binge eating, which—guess what?—leads to more weight gain.

483. ▪ **Limit your carbohydrates to the level that is best for you.** Carbohydrate and sugar tolerance lessens with age and varies from individual to individual. For most people, a moderate intake of roughly 40 percent carbohydrates in their diets is more appropriate for health than a high-carbohydrate intake. Remember that too many carbohydrates in your system can lead to high levels of insulin, the fat-storage hormone. High insulin levels are not only probable precursors of obesity, but also of heart disease, diabetes, and numerous other serious health conditions.

484. ▪ **An overlooked key to weight control** is maintaining a steady blood-sugar level. Eating high-glycemic foods such as sugar may initially give you fast peaks in energy, but it will also cause a fast fall in blood sugar and energy that will leave you wanting more sugar later on. To maintain your blood sugar in the optimal zone for weight control, long-term energy, and health, emphasize instead low- and moderate-glycemic foods, foods that are as close to their natural state as possible, and a balance of high-quality protein, fat, and carbohydrates.

485. ▪ **Get back to basics if you want to lose weight.** If you think about it, the most obvious and the safest way to promote weight loss is to avoid foods that give you unnecessary calories. Sugars, processed carbohydrates, and alcohol—which give you little of the nutrients you require—are the top three on that list.

486. ▪ **If you have tried every diet that there is** and have never experienced any permanent weight loss, understand that you need to give up the dieting game and adopt a sensible low-sugar eating plan for life. If you don't believe a lifelong low-sugar plan will benefit you in countless ways, I challenge you to try limiting the grains you consume to two servings per day and eating no more than twenty grams of sugar per day for one month. If you try this experiment, you might just be amazed at how your body responds.

THE REST OF THE WORLD

487. ▪ **Try going on a buddy system** with a friend who is also trying to cut the sugar out. The support and camaraderie from someone else in your shoes is often immeasurable.

488. ▪ **Or hire your own special buddy—a qualified nutritionist**—to help you with the practical ups and downs common with giving up sugar. A health professional trained in nutrition can assist you with both the biochemical and emotional aspects of getting the sugar out as well as develop an individualized plan just for you.

489. ▪ **Be diplomatic but honest with your friends and relatives** and tell them that you would appreciate their not bringing sweets or spoiling your children with treats anymore. In a pleasant way, make it clear to them what you will allow and why you feel that way, and you might even get them to start thinking about going on their own sugar-lowering adventures!

490. ▪ **Also check with your children's day-care providers and teachers** and make sure that sugar is not being used, as it often is, to pacify, reward, or discipline your children. Explain your feelings and most people will honor and respect them.

491. ▪ **Don't ever offer your child a sweet treat as a reward** to get him or her to eat. Doing so sets up an unhealthy situation and an even greater desire to indulge that sweet tooth.

492. ▪ **Prevent babies from developing an excessive sweet tooth** by not giving them nursing bottles full of fruit juice or water with honey or sugar in it. Giving children sweet drinks early in life sets the stage for tooth decay and promotes a strong desire for sweets that can lead to obesity later on.

493. ▪ **Enlist the assistance of your children** to help you find acceptable foods at the grocery store. Children are often willing to help, and if you make a game out of reading labels and finding good foods, they usually have fun responding to the challenge. They also learn a lot about food, and how much sugar there is in food.

494. ▪ **Be creative when packing your school-age children's lunches.** Try to provide your children with healthful, fun, and nourishing treats that look so good their friends will want them, too. The more you can accomplish this, the more your children will relish eating what you packed and not resort to the overly sweet, tooth-demolishing, mass-produced junk food available at so many schools today.

495. ▪ **All in the family? Why not?** Try to get others in your family to kick the sugar habit with you. It's much easier to stay away from sugar when the people close to you will also. Even if they won't, be sure they understand and respect just how important avoiding sugar is to you.

▪ ▪ ▪

HEALTHY ATTITUDES, HEALTHY LIFE

496. ▪ **Refrain from getting discouraged and persevere,** even when it seems as if all the people in the world (including your closest friends) are indulging their sweet tooth. You have to understand that you now know a secret many have yet to learn: Limiting your sugar intake is the key to better-looking skin, balanced moods, concentration, a trim physique, less illness, and better all-around health. I myself find it much easier to go against the grain and keep the sugar out of my diet because I know that my efforts are paying off in how I look and feel today and will in the future.

497. ▪ **Concentrate on changing yourself for the better,** even when others close to you are not interested in doing the same. When others see how helpful getting the sugar out is for you, they might just follow your lead. Even if they don't, you need to remember that your primary responsibility in life is to be the best person that you can possibly be.

498. ▪ **Picture yourself being easily in control of the sugar you consume** and having a balanced, healthy attitude to food in general. Positive visualizations often translate into positive results.

499. ▪ **To ensure success, reinforce your commitment to eat for health** as much as you need. One person I know who had severe immune dysfunction posted this affirmation on her refrigerator to help her lick her sugar habit: "I want and deserve to take good care of myself. I can pass up sugar and be totally happy about it because I am replacing temporary, short-lived satisfaction in exchange for the greater satisfaction of long-term, radiant health." (This meditation that she saw every day obviously worked. The woman is now free of her immunity problems.)

500. ▪ **Value yourself enough to nourish yourself with life-giving whole food.** Certain cultures, such as some Native American tribes and the Chinese, believe that both plant-based and animal-based whole foods have a life force that strengthens our own life force when we eat them. When foods such as wheat and sugar are refined, however, the natural balance of minerals in these foods is destroyed, and they no longer supply the nutrition and the supportive energy they once did. Understanding this, you can choose unrefined foods over refined ones and take an important step toward better physical health and, consequently, better emotional, mental, and spiritual health as well.

501. ▪ **Treat yourself often to sweet experiences** in place of sweet food. Give yourself license to enjoy forgotten-about pleasures that don't revolve around food, such as soaking in fragrant herbal baths; getting a relaxing massage; communing with nature; listening to uplifting music; buying yourself a long-awaited piece of clothing; or reading an adventure novel that takes you away for a while. When you allow yourself these kinds of healthy indulgences, sugar treats no longer seem necessary or desirable.

AFTERWORD

arlier in my career, I went against traditional dietary wisdom when I wrote my first book, *Beyond Pritikin*. In that book, I explained how the right type of fat should not be avoided but rather included in the diet to promote optimal health. Now that health-conscious consumers such as you are starting to comprehend this message, it's high time you learn the equally important message that *sugar should be avoided* because it is, without a doubt, hazardous to human health. This book was written to remind you of this overlooked information and to show you practical ways to put this knowledge to work for you.

Facing up to the truth about sugar has not always been easy for me. I myself used to binge on sugar. I also know all too well how hard it is to avoid a substance that the rest of America holds in such high esteem.

But I had to start seeing the truth about sugar when my own father was diagnosed with adult-onset diabetes. Since there is a history of diabetes in my family and since diseases such as diabetes are linked to excessive sugar intake, I gradually began to realize that I had to get the sugar out of my diet to ensure my best health for the future.

More and more people are coming to this same conclusion. The evidence against sugar is simply too overwhelming to ignore.

Since you now know that eating too much sugar is tied to the most widespread and devastating illnesses of this century, act on what you know and limit your sugar consumption as the best way to maintain your health.

Sugar is not talked about much right now as the villain it truly is, but I promise you that this will change. As more research continues to uncover insulin's role in disease—and as more Americans see that their fat-free experiment is not working—the dangers of excessive sugar in the diet will be emphasized.

Our society will eventually catch up with current information about sugar, but until it does, be a trailblazer and use your knowledge for a healthy edge.

APPENDIX

Here is a weeklong sample menu that incorporates the topics covered in *Get the Sugar Out*. The menu is designed to give you an idea of some of the things you can eat on a low-sugar eating plan for life.

As you can see, when you're on a health-maintenance diet such as this one, deprivation does not enter into the picture. You can have a wide variety of delicious food—even such treats as Danish pastries, cookies, and ice cream—as long as you choose your treats intelligently and incorporate them into a balanced diet.

This plan emphasizes the natural sugars in fresh vegetables and fruits and keeps the grams of sugars to between twenty and forty a day. *Any level below forty grams is a good goal for all of us to shoot for.*

If, however, you are having trouble losing weight—or if you are recovering from diabetes, heart disease, cancer, parasites, yeast problems, or other health conditions—you should consider reducing sugars to below twenty grams per day. This level seems to allow maximum healing to take place and can be accomplished by substituting a serving of a low-starch vegetable (listed in tip 240) in place of any dessert or fruit listed on the menu.

This plan is just one example of how you can put the tips from this book into practice. The key to successful low-sugar eating is to use the sugar savvy you have learned to create a personal program that works for you.

▪ **MONDAY** ▪

Breakfast—2 Almond-Oat Granola Squares (tip 280)

Lunch—Salad plate with 1 cup romaine lettuce, $\frac{1}{2}$ cup
mixed baby greens, shredded red cabbage and carrot, and
chopped tomato and cucumber
Topped with 3 ounces of broiled seasoned chicken-breast strips
and 2 tablespoons vinegar-and-oil dressing

Dinner—Baked turkey meatballs made with 4 ounces ground
turkey, oat bran, chopped onion, marjoram, and parsley
1 serving Spaghetti Squash Italian (tip 222) with Pasta Sauce
(tip 250)

▪ **TUESDAY** ▪

Breakfast—$\frac{1}{2}$ cup low-fat cottage cheese
$\frac{1}{4}$ cantaloupe (6-inch diameter)

Lunch—1 bean burrito made with $\frac{1}{2}$ cup mashed pinto beans and
1 whole-wheat tortilla
Topped with chopped tomato, onion, and shredded lettuce,
$\frac{1}{2}$ tablespoon guacamole with no sugar added, and
1 tablespoon salsa with no sugar added

Dinner—4 ounces broiled shrimp marinated in sesame oil, lime
juice, garlic, and coriander
$\frac{1}{2}$ cup spelt pasta
Topped with $\frac{1}{2}$ cup zucchini, asparagus, and green onion
sautéed in sesame or olive oil with fresh basil
1 baked Vanilla Pear (tip 343) *or* $\frac{1}{2}$ cup fresh pineapple tidbits
topped with 1 tablespoon unsweetened shredded coconut

▪ WEDNESDAY ▪

Breakfast—1 hard-boiled egg
$\frac{1}{2}$ cup Crock-Pot Rye Cereal (tip 147) *or* 1 slice of sourdough rye toast

Lunch—1 Peanut Butter and Apple Sandwich with 2 tablespoons unsweetened peanut butter and thin slices of 1 fresh apple on 2 slices whole-grain bread

Dinner—1 serving Five-Spice Chicken and Vegetable Sauté, with broccoli, red pepper, carrots, yellow squash, onion, and water chestnuts (tip 234)
$\frac{1}{2}$ cup brown rice
$\frac{3}{4}$ cup sliced fresh strawberries topped with a dollop of low-fat cultured yogurt mixed with a pinch of FOS (tip 344) and a dash of natural vanilla extract (tip 345)

▪ THURSDAY ▪

Breakfast—1 Mock Danish Pastry (tip 121) *or*
2 toasted Whole-Grain Pumpkin Muffins (tip 118) spread with 1 tablespoon Peach Butter (tip 111), 1 tablespoon Carrot Butter (tip 112), *or* 1 teaspoon cinnamon-sprinkled butter (tip 105)

Lunch—Tuna salad made with 3 ounces of canned tuna, celery, green onion tops, water chestnuts, fresh lemon juice, and $\frac{1}{2}$ tablespoon canola mayonnaise
Served on Bibb lettuce or spinach leaves

Dinner—Roast Cornish game hen sprinkled with sage or thyme
$\frac{1}{2}$ cup mixed green peas and carrots
$\frac{1}{2}$ cup brussels sprouts with 1 teaspoon butter

▪ **FRIDAY** ▪

Breakfast—½ cup oatmeal with 1 tablespoon raisins, 2 tablespoons chopped walnuts, and a sprinkling of ground cinnamon
½ cup nonfat milk
1 cup French Vanilla Café (tip 162)

Lunch—Hamburger made out of ¼ pound broiled ground round
Served on a whole-grain spelt bun with lettuce, tomato, red-onion slices, and 1 teaspoon horseradish-spiked Dijon mustard
5 small jicama sticks

Dinner—3 ounces baked sole brushed with 1 teaspoon olive oil and fresh dill, served with a lemon wedge
1 cup green beans almondine
3 small Oatmeal–Chocolate Chip Cookies (tip 396) *or* 1 serving Chocolate Ice Cream (tip 424)

▪ **SATURDAY** ▪

Breakfast—2 poached eggs on 1 slice toasted 12-grain bread
½ grapefruit

Lunch—1 cup lentil soup with no sugar added
1 serving Butternut Squash Pudding (tip 352)

Dinner—3 ounces roast turkey-breast slices au jus
1 small cooked sweet potato with 1 teaspoon butter
½ cup steamed broccoli and cauliflower

▪ **SUNDAY** ▪

Brunch—5 Homemade Turkey Sausage patties (tip 140)
6 Melissa's Sweet Potato Pancakes (tip 129) topped with ¼ cup unsweetened peach applesauce

Snack—1 Pizza Muffin (tip 272)
2 carrot strips and 2 celery sticks
10 large fresh cherries

Dinner—4 ounces broiled lamb chops with garlic, oregano, and lemon
⅓ cup long-grain brown rice, wild rice, and mushroom medley
Side salad with red leaf lettuce, chopped tomato, cucumber, and 1 tablespoon French Olive Oil Dressing (tip 191)

Note: Remember to avoid sugars in the drinks you consume throughout the day. Choose any of the following sugar-free beverages both with meals and as mini-refreshers between meals: filtered water, mineral water, sparkling water, herbal teas, stevia-sweetened drinks, and FOS-sweetened drinks.

RESOURCES

AATRON MEDICAL SERVICES
12832 S. Chadron Avenue
Hawthorne, CA 90250
1-800-367-7744
1-800-433-9750 (in California)

A laboratory that specializes in testing the levels of amino acids by analyzing plasma and urine samples. Will also provide courtesy consultations with clients over the phone.

ALLERGY RESOURCES
P.O. Box 888
Palmer Lake, CO 80133
1-719-488-3630
1-800-USE-FLAX

A mail order company that sells a wide selection of natural and alternative food and health products, including hard-to-find food items mentioned in this book such as maple syrup granules, date "sugar," fructose, FOS (fructooligosaccharides), and stevia. Call for a free catalog.

AMERICAN ACADEMY OF NUTRITION
1200 Kenesaw
Knoxville, TN 37919-7736
1-800-290-4226

The American Academy of Nutrition offers more than twenty nutrition home-study courses, as well as a recently developed associate-of-science degree program in applied nutrition. This institution is the only home-study nutrition education school in the world that is accredited by the U.S. Department of Education's Distance Education Training Council. Ann Louise Gittleman serves as the director of continuing education for the academy and recommends the academy's courses for anyone wishing to become more knowledgeable about the important subject of human nutrition.

B.E.D. PUBLICATIONS
(The Body Ecology Diet)
1266 West Paces Ferry Road, Suite 505
Atlanta, GA 30327
1-800-4-STEVIA (478-3842)

The Body Ecology Company sells stevia and also supplies hard-to-find sweet-tasting recipes that use stevia.

UNI-KEY HEALTH SYSTEMS
P.O. Box 7168
Bozeman, MT 59771
1-800-888-4353

Uni-Key is a mail order company that sells innovative natural products to Ann Louise's clients and readers. Be sure to use Uni-Key if you have trouble finding quality supplements that will assist you in getting the sugar out or if you have difficulty locating any of Ann Louise's books.

BIBLIOGRAPHY

Abrahamson, E. M., M.D., and A. W. Pezet. *Body, Mind and Sugar.* New York: Holt, Rinehart and Winston, 1951.

Allman, William F. "Aspartame: Some Bitter with the Sweet?" *Science* 84, 5 (July/August 1984): 14.

Appleton, Nancy. *Lick the Sugar Habit.* Garden City Park, N.Y.: Avery Publishing Group, 1988.

Atkins, Robert C., M.D. *Dr. Atkins' New Diet Revolution.* New York: M. Evans and Company, 1992.

Barkie, Karen E. *Sweet and Sugarfree.* New York: St. Martin's Press, 1982.

Blaylock, Russell, M.D. *Excitotoxins: The Taste That Kills.* Santa Fe, N.M.: Health Press, 1994.

Blumenthal, Mark. "Is Stevia Too Sweet for Us?" *Let's Live,* June 1992, 66–67.

Buhr, Deborah E. *The "I Can't Believe This Has No Sugar" Cookbook.* New York: St. Martin's Press, 1990.

Burrows, Nancy. *Allergy Cooking Tricks and Treasures.* Grand Forks, N.D.: Nancy Burrows, 1987.

Cleave, T. L. *The Saccharine Disease.* New Canaan, Conn.: Keats Publishing, 1975.

"The Confectionery Elite 1994." *Confectioner,* May/June 1995.

Crayhon, Robert, M.S. *Health Benefits of FOS (Fructooligosaccharides).* New Canaan, Conn.: Keats Publishing, 1995.

———. *Robert Crayhon's Nutrition Made Simple.* New York: M. Evans and Company, 1994.

Crook, William G., M.D., and Marjorie Hurt Jones, R.N. *The Yeast Connection Cookbook.* Jackson, Tenn.: Professional Books, 1989.

Crook, William G., M.D. *The Yeast Connection and the Woman.* Jackson, Tenn.: Professional Books, 1995.

Dufty, William. *Sugar Blues.* New York: Warner Books, 1975.

Dumke, Nicolette M. *Allergy Cooking with Ease.* Lancaster, Pa.: Starburst Publishers, 1992.

———. "Stevia, the Herbal Sweetener." *Mastering Food Allergies,* April 1991, 1–2.

Fallon, Sally W., B.A. "Fructose Folly." *PPNF Health Journal* 19, no. 1 (Spring 1995): 4–6.

Fredericks, Carlton, and Herman Goodman, M.D. *Low Blood Sugar and You.* New York: Grosset and Dunlap, 1969.

Galland, Leo, M.D. *Super Immunity for Kids.* New York: Copestone Press, Inc., 1988.

Gates, Donna. *The Body Ecology Diet.* Atlanta, Ga.: B.E.D. Publications, 1993.

Gerras, Charles, ed., and the staff of Rodale Press. *Rodale's Basic Natural Foods Cookbook.* New York: Rodale Press, 1984.

Gittleman, Ann Louise, M.S. *Beyond Pritikin.* New York: Bantam Books, 1996.

———. *Super Nutrition for Menopause.* New York: Pocket Books, 1993.

———. *Super Nutrition for Women.* New York: Bantam Books, 1991.

———. *Your Body Knows Best.* New York: Pocket Books, 1996.

Goldbeck, Nikki and David. *The Good Breakfast Book.* Woodstock, N.Y.: Ceres Press, 1992.

Hunt, Douglas, M.D. *No More Cravings.* New York: Warner Books, 1987.

Jones, Jeanne. *Cook It Light.* New York: Macmillan Publishing Company, 1987.

Jones, Marjorie Hurt, R.N. *The Allergy Self-Help Cookbook.* Emmaus, Pa.: Rodale Books, 1984.

Kamen, Betty, Ph.D. *The Chromium Diet, Supplement & Exercise Strategy.* Novato, Calif.: Nutrition Encounter, Inc., 1990.

Kinderlehrer, Jane. *Smart Breakfasts.* New York: Newmarket Press, 1989.

———. *Smart Chicken.* New York: Newmarket Press, 1991.

———. *Smart Cookies.* New York: Newmarket Press, 1991.

———. *Smart Muffins.* New York: Newmarket Press, 1987.

Krohn, Jacqueline, M.D., et al. *The Whole Way to Allergy Relief and Prevention.* Point Roberts, Wash.: Hartley & Marks, Inc., 1991.

Kuczmarski, Robert J., Dr.PH., R.D., et al. "Increasing Prevalence of Overweight Among U.S. Adults." *Journal of the American Medical Association* 272 (1994): 205–11.

Leahy, Linda Romanelli. *The All-Natural Sugar-Free Dessert Cookbook.* New York: Dell Publishing, 1992.

Mason, Michael. "Confessions of a Fat-Free Snack Junkie." *Health*, May/June 1995, 36, 42.

Melos, Linda. *Sugar and Carbohydrate Intolerance.* Phoenix, Ariz.: Eck Institute reference sheet, 1987.

Mindell, Earl, Ph.D. *Safe Eating.* New York: Warner Books, 1987.

Nostrand, Carol A. *Junk Food to Real Food.* New Canaan, Conn.: Keats Publishing, 1994.

O'Neill, Molly. "So It May Be True After All: Eating Pasta Makes You Fat." *New York Times*, February 8, 1995.

Quillin, Patrick, Ph.D., R.D. *Beating Cancer with Nutrition.* Tulsa, Okla.: The Nutrition Times Press, 1994.

Phelps, Janice Keller, M.D., and Allan E. Nourse, M.D. *The Hidden Addiction and How to Get Free.* Boston: Little, Brown and Company, 1986.

Pitchford, Paul. *Healing with Whole Foods.* Berkeley, Calif.: North Atlantic Books, 1993.

Rector-Page, Linda. *Cooking for Healthy Healing.* Sonora, Calif.: Healthy Healing Publications, 1991.

Remington, Dennis W., M.D., and Barbara W. Higa, R.D. *Back to Health.* Provo, Utah: Vitality House International, Inc., 1986.

Roth, Harriet. *Deliciously Low*. New York: New American Library, 1983.

Schauss, Alexander. *Diet, Crime and Delinquency*. Berkeley, Calif.: Parker House, 1981.

Schauss, Alexander, et al. *Eating for A's*. New York: Pocket Books, 1991.

Spiller, Gene, M.D. *The Superpyramid Eating Program*. New York: Random House, 1993.

Townsley, Cheryl. *Kids' Favorites*. Littleton, Colo.: Cheryl Townsley, 1992.

Warrington, Janet. *Sweet and Natural*. Freedom, Calif.: The Crossing Press, 1982.

Yudkin, John, M.D. *Sweet and Dangerous*. New York: Wyden Books, 1972.

PERMISSIONS

"Almond Milkshake" from *Healing with Whole Foods: Oriental Traditions and Modern Nutrition,* by Paul Pitchford. Copyright © 1993, 1996 by Paul Pitchford. Reprinted by permission of Atlantic Books, Berkeley, California.

"Amaretto Cheesecake Tarts" adapted from *Smart Cookies* by Jane Kinderlehrer. Copyright © 1985 by Jane Kinderlehrer. Reprinted by permission of Newmarket Press, 18 East 48th Street, New York, New York 10017.

"Baked Sweet Beans" from *Healing with Whole Foods: Oriental Traditions and Modern Nutrition,* by Paul Pitchford. Copyright © 1993, 1996 by Paul Pitchford. Reprinted by permission of Atlantic Books, Berkeley, California.

"Butternut Bisque" reprinted with the permission of Simon & Schuster from *Super Nutrition for Menopause* by Ann Louise Gittleman. Copyright © 1993 by Ann Louise Gittleman, MS.

"California Guacamole Dressing" from *Cooking for Healthy Healing,* by Linda Rector-Page. Copyright © 1995 by Linda Rector-Page. Reprinted by permission of Healthy Healing Publications/Crystal Star.

"Carob or Chocolate Frosting" from *Kid Smart: Raising a Healthy Child* by Cheryl Townsley. Copyright © 1992 by Cheryl Townsley. Reproduced by permission of LFH Publications.

Gittleman. Copyright © 1988 by Ann Louise Gittleman. Reprinted by permission of Bantam Books, a division of Bantam Doubleday Dell Publishing Group, Inc.

"Fresh Pasta Sauce." Reprinted by permission of Holly J. Sollars.

"Fruity Tofu Delight." Reprinted by permission of Holly J. Sollars.

"Green Herb Sauce." Copyright © 1996 by Gene Spiller. From *Eat Your Way to Better Health,* Prima Publishing, Rocklin, CA. Call 800-632-8676.

"Homemade Turkey Sausage." Reprinted by permission of Melissa Diane Smith.

"Last Minute Fruit Melange." Copyright © 1983 by Harriet Roth from *Deliciously Low* by Harriet Roth. Used by permission of Dutton Signet, a division of Penguin Books USA, Inc.

"Lemon or Cranberry Cooler" from *The Body Ecology Diet* by Donna Gates. Copyright © 1993 by Donna Gates. Reprinted by permission of Donna Gates.

"Magic Apple Pie" adapted from *The Yeast Connection Cookbook* by William G. Crook, M.D., and Marjorie Hurt Jones. Copyright © 1989 by William G. Crook, M.D., and Marjorie Hurt Jones. Reprinted by permission of Professional Books.

"Melissa's Sweet Potato Pancakes." Reprinted by permission of Melissa Diane Smith.

"Mock Danish Pastry" from *Eating for A's* by Alexander Schauss, et al. Copyright © 1991 by Alexander Schauss, et al. Reprinted by permission of the authors.

"No-Bake Cheese Pie" adapted from *Rodale's Basic Natural Foods Cookbook.* Copyright © 1983 by Rodale Press, Inc. Reprinted by permission of Rodale Press, Inc., Emmaus, PA 18098.

"Oat Granola" from *The Yeast Connection Cookbook* by William G. Crook, M.D. and Marjorie Hurt Jones. Copyright © 1989 by William G. Crook, M.D. and Majorie Hurt Jones. Reprinted by permission of Professional Books.

"Oatmeal–Chocolate Chip Cookies." Reprinted by permission of Melissa Diane Smith.

INDEX